Ethnic and Global Perspectives to Facial Plastic Surgery

Editors

ROXANA COBO
ANTHONY E. BRISSETT
KOFI BOAHENE

FACIAL PLASTIC SURGERY CLINICS OF NORTH AMERICA

www.facialplastic.theclinics.com

Consulting Editor
J. REGAN THOMAS

November 2022 • Volume 30 • Number 4

ELSEVIER

1600 John F. Kennedy Boulevard • Suite 1800 • Philadelphia, Pennsylvania, 19103-2899

http://www.theclinics.com

FACIAL PLASTIC SURGERY CLINICS OF NORTH AMERICA Volume 30, Number 4
November 2022 ISSN 1064-7406, ISBN-13: 978-0-323-97298-7

Editor: Stacy Eastman
Developmental Editor: Ann Gielou M. Posedio

Facial Plastic Surgery Clinics of North America (ISSN 1064-7406) is published quarterly by Elsevier Inc., 360 Park Avenue South, New York, NY 10010-1710. Months of issue are February, May, August, and November. Business and Editorial Offices: 1600 John F. Kennedy Blvd., Suite 1800, Philadelphia, PA 19103-2899. Periodicals postage paid at New York, NY, and additional mailing offices. Subscription prices are $420.00 per year (US individuals), $922.00 per year (US institutions), $468.00 per year (Canadian individuals), $950.00 per year (Canadian institutions), $557.00 per year (foreign individuals), $950.00 per year (foreign institutions), $100.00 per year (US students), $100.00 per year (Canadian students), and $255.00 per year (foreign students). Foreign air speed delivery is included in all *Clinics* subscription prices. All prices are subject to change without notice. POSTMASTER: Send address changes to *Facial Plastic Surgery Clinics*, Elsevier Health Sciences Division, Subscription Customer Service, 3251 Riverport Lane, Maryland Heights, MO 63043. **Customer service: 1-800-654-2452 (US and Canada); 1-314-447-8871 (outside US and Canada); Fax: 314-447-8029; E-mail: journalscustomerservice-usa@elsevier.com (for print support); journalsonlinesupport-usa@elsevier.com (for online support).**

Reprints. For copies of 100 or more of articles in this publication, please contact the Commercial Reprints Department, Elsevier Inc., 360 Park Avenue South, New York, NY 10010-1710. Tel.: 212-633-3874; Fax: 212-633-3820; E-mail: reprints@elsevier.com.

Facial Plastic Surgery Clinics of North America is covered in *MEDLINE/PubMed* (*Index Medicus*).

Contributors

CONSULTING EDITOR

J. REGAN THOMAS, MD
Professor, Facial Plastic and Reconstructive Surgery, Department of Otolaryngology–Head and Neck Surgery, Northwestern University Feinberg School of Medicine, Chicago, Illinois

EDITORS

ROXANA COBO, MD
Chief, Department of Otorhinolaryngology, Private Practice, Facial Plastic Surgery, Clinica Imbanaco, Cali, Colombia

ANTHONY E. BRISSETT, MD, FACS
Professor and Vice Chair, Department of Otolaryngoglogy–Head and Neck Surgery, Division Chief, Division of Facial Plastic and Reconstructive Surgery, Houston Methodist Hospital, Weill Cornell College of Medicine, Houston Methodist ENT Specialists, Houston, Texas, USA

KOFI BOAHENE, MD
Professor and Chief, Division of Facial Plastic and Reconstructive Surgery, Johns Hopkins School of Medicine, Johns Hopkins Facial Plastic and Reconstructive Surgery Center, Lutherville, Maryland, USA; Professor, Otolaryngology–Head and Neck Surgery, Division of Facial Plastic and Reconstructive Surgery, Johns Hopkins School of Medicine, Johns Hopkins Outpatient Center, Baltimore, Maryland, USA

AUTHORS

ABDURRAHMAN "ABDUL" AL-AWADY, BS
University of Miami Miller School of Medicine, MD Class of 2023

PETER A. ADAMSON, OONT, MD, FRCSC, FACS
Professor, Division of Facial Plastic and Reconstructive Surgery, Department of Otolaryngology–Head and Neck Surgery, University of Toronto, Toronto, Ontario, Canada

KOFI BOAHENE, MD
Professor and Chief, Division of Facial Plastic and Reconstructive Surgery, Johns Hopkins School of Medicine, Johns Hopkins Facial Plastic and Reconstructive Surgery Center, Lutherville, Maryland, USA; Professor, Otolaryngology–Head and Neck Surgery, Division of Facial Plastic and Reconstructive Surgery, Johns Hopkins School of Medicine, Johns Hopkins Outpatient Center, Baltimore, Maryland, USA

ANTHONY E. BRISSETT, MD, FACS
Professor and Vice Chair, Department of Otolaryngoglogy–Head and Neck Surgery, Division Chief, Division of Facial Plastic and Reconstructive Surgery, Houston Methodist Hospital, Weill Cornell College of Medicine, Houston Methodist ENT Specialists, Houston, Texas, USA

ÖZCAN ÇAKMAK, MD
Professor, European Board-Certified Facial Plastic Surgeon, FACEISTANBUL, Private Practice, Istanbul, Turkey

JUAN GABRIEL CAMACHO TRIANA, MD
Otolaryngologist, Bogota, Colombia

MIRIAM DE LA TORRE CAMPOS, MD
Otolaryngology, Facial Plastic Surgeon, Private
Practice and Professor, Department of
Otolaryngology Facial Plastic Surgery, Hospital
San Jose de Hermosillo, Hermosillo, Sonora,
Mexico

ROXANA COBO, MD
Chief, Department of Otorhinolaryngology,
Private Practice, Facial Plastic Surgery, Clinica
Imbanaco, Cali, Colombia

RAFAEL ESPINOSA DELGADO, MD
Otolaryngology, Facial Plastic Surgeon, Private
Practice and Professor, Department of
Otolaryngology Facial Plastic Surgery, Hospital
San Jose de Hermosillo, Hermosillo, Sonora,
Mexico, Past President of the Mexican Society
of Facial Plastic Surgery and Rhinology

**DAVID EDWARD JAMES WHITEHEAD,
MBBS, BSC, MSC, FRCS(ORL-HNS)**
Visiting Fellow, FACEISTANBUL, Istanbul,
Turkey

GORANA KUKA EPSTEIN, MD
Voluntary Professor, Voluntary Assistant
Professor, Philip Frost Department of
Dermatology and Cutaneous Surgery,
University of Miami Miller School of Medicine

JEFFREY S. EPSTEIN, MD, FACS
Voluntary Professor, Voluntary Assistant
Professor, Philip Frost Department of
Dermatology and Cutaneous Surgery,
Department of Otolaryngology, University of
Miami Miller School of Medicine

JORGE A. ESPINOSA REYES, MD
Otolaryngologist, Facial Plastic Surgeon,
Bogota, Colombia

TANG HO, MD, MSC
Associate Professor, Chief of Facial Plastic and
Reconstructive Surgery, Department of

Otorhinolaryngology–Head and Neck Surgery,
Texas Center for Facial Plastic Surgery,
McGovern Medical School, The University of
Texas Health Science Center in Houston,
Houston, Texas, USA

YONG JU JANG, MD, PhD
Department of Otorhinolaryngology–Head and
Neck Surgery, Asan Medical Center, University
of Ulsan College of Medicine, Songpa-gu,
Seoul, Republic of Korea

W. KATHERINE KAO, MD
Assistant Professor, Department of
Otorhinolaryngology–Head and Neck Surgery,
Texas Center for Facial Plastic Surgery,
McGovern Medical School, The University of
Texas Health Science Center in Houston,
Houston, Texas, USA

SEAN P. MCKEE, MD
Department of Otorhinolaryngology–Head and
Neck Surgery, McGovern Medical School, The
University of Texas Health Science Center at
Houston, Houston, Texas, USA

**AMANI A. OBEID, MBBS, SB-ORL HNS,
FACS**
Facial Plastic and Reconstructive Surgery
Consultant, Department of Otolaryngology,
Head and Neck Surgery, King Saud University,
King Saud University Medical City, Riyadh,
Saudi Arabia

MARN JOON PARK, MD
Department of Otorhinolaryngology–Head and
Neck Surgery, Asan Medical Center, University
of Ulsan College of Medicine, Songpa-gu,
Seoul, Republic of Korea

BLAKE S. RAGGIO, MD
Alabama Plastic and Reconstructive Surgery,
Jackson Hospital and Clinics, Montgomery,
Alabama, USA

Contents

> Beauty is a mystical and powerful, indeed existential, force. Beauty can be described philosophically, quantified mathematically, and defined biologically. Our individual attractiveness confers real benefits and impacts our reproductive success. Natural beauty is perceived similarly by all races and cultures yet has unique ethnic characteristics. Various artificial beauty interventions are used across all cultures to enhance natural beauty. The forces of globalization, especially social media and even the pandemic, are accelerating the evolution of attractiveness and beauty standards worldwide. Future neuropsychiatric and biopsychological interventions may allow us to change how we perceive beauty in ourselves and others.

> Mixed-race patients seeking noninvasive esthetic procedures with minimal to no downtime are increasing, the most common issue in this group of patients when using medical technologies is post-inflammatory hyperpigmentation or hypopigmentation. Radiofrequency (RF) is an energy that is safe for treating all skin types because it does not interact target chromophore, its mechanism of action is the production of heat by shooting electrons into tissue and the interaction with that tissue's impedance or resistance is what produces the heat, and the heat induces collagen remodeling and collagenesis, so skin color, melanin, and hemoglobin do not play any role in RF-based treatments.

> Hair restoration surgery is a popular procedure among patients of all ethnic groups. Whether performing hair procedures to treat male and female pattern hair loss, or to restore eyebrows and beards, or to shorten overly high hairlines, the surgeon must consider differences in esthetic ideals, hair characteristics, and healing properties to achieve optimal results.

> The Asian eyelid has distinct anatomic features that distinguish it from the Caucasian eyelid. These anatomic features are responsible for the ethnic identity of the Asian

eyelid and guide operative technique and intervention. In the younger patient, the goal of Asian blepharoplasty often centers on the enhancement of the ethnic eye features and the creation of the supratarsal fold often referred to as the "double eyelid." In the aging Asian eyelid, considerations should be made to evaluate and address dermatochalasis, blepharoptosis, and brow ptosis. In patients with significant lateral brow ptosis and lateral hooding, the infrabrow excision blepharoplasty technique may provide an additional functional and esthetic benefit.

  Video content accompanies this article at http://www.facialplastic.theclinics.com.

In this article, we present the anatomy, diagnosis, surgical technique, and postoperative care of the buccal fat pad removal. Anatomy knowledge and careful surgical technique are the primary considerations for a successful procedure with a low incidence of complications. The technique's main characteristics are the intraoral approach using blunt dissection and suction-assisted buccal fat pad extraction.

Despite the propensity for humans to classify themselves into separate ethnoraces, the stigma of aging eventually appears in all. The mobile superficial musculoaponeurotic system is a key area of change across all ethnicities and can be rejuvenated most effectively when the cutaneous retaining ligaments of the face and neck are fully released. The extended facelift techniques are logically the most effective in achieving this. Despite facelift surgery, the neck is often neglected but can be managed in a variety of ways. Changes within the deep neck structures are most effectively addressed under direct vision through a midline submental incision.

The zygomaticomaxillary complex and mandible play a significant role in facial beauty. The projection of these bones drapes and conforms the overlying soft tissues, resulting in the light reflections and shadows that define a face. The size, contour, and projection of these bones of beauty are sexually dimorphic and ethnically defined. Excessive projection of these bones in any dimension can lead to undesirable esthetic appearance. Reduction malarplasty and mandibuloplasty are effective techniques that can be used to reshape the facial skeleton to a more desirable shape.

In this article 2 rhinoplasty cases involving patients of African descent are presented. One of these highlights the correction of a dorsal contour irregularity and an amorphous and ptotic tip with a widened alar base, addressed through an open approach. The second case focuses on improving nasal tip definition through an endonasal approach.

Today, primary rhinoplasty in Latino patients is tailored based on a targeted approach depending on the individual patient's needs and desires. The goal always is to achieve stable long-term results. This article presents 2 types of patients undergoing primary rhinoplasty: a patient with a small hump or "pseudo" osteocartilaginous hump that was treated using a hybrid approach (surface dorsal preservation technique) and a patient with a low nasal dorsum that was augmented using a diced cartilage glue graft. In both cases the nasal tips had poor structure and flimsy support and were treated using different structural grafting techniques.

 Video content accompanies this article at http://www.facialplastic.theclinics.com.

The increased popularity of rhinoplasty in the Middle East has been observed in the last decade among all age groups. The ideal nasal shape varies widely between different Middle Eastern countries, and sometimes even within different regions in the same country. This article discusses a case study on these variations and beauty ideals, which a rhinoplasty surgeon should be aware of.

To achieve an esthetically satisfying surgical outcome in rhinoplasty of East Asians, it is most important to emphasize the augmentation of the flattened nose. However, correction of the accompanying nasal deviation or hump reduction together with appropriate tip work is essential for a successful outcome following rhinoplasty. Additionally, the surgeon must be aware of cosmetic deformities following silicone rhinoplasty and should be capable of appropriate nasal reconstruction in patients with silicone implant-related problems.

FACIAL PLASTIC SURGERY CLINICS OF NORTH AMERICA

THE CLINICS ARE AVAILABLE ONLINE!
Access your subscription at:
www.theclinics.com

Foreword
The Principles and Practice of Beauty

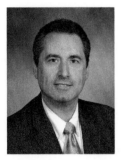

Anthony P. Sclafani, MD, MBA, FACS

When discussing the concept of "beauty," it is important to take a critical look at one's biases, preferences, cultural background, and social position, among other things. We bring to the discussion our own attitudes, formed over decades through our environment, upbringing, and experiences. If our purpose as facial plastic surgeons is to help patients define and achieve a particular goal as to their appearance, we must understand how that goal fits into the larger "definition" of beauty.

As the world becomes more interconnected and communities become less insular, facial plastic surgeons need to broaden our perspectives and our viewpoints to better relate to our patients and understand their goals. Neoclassical canons of beauty, developed over centuries and promulgated widely throughout the last 500 years, are based on a rather narrow selection of ideals. These canons do not represent the full spectrum of our patients. The diligent surgeon does not rely on a single conceptualization of beauty; rather, the enlightened surgeon learns the factors that determine facial form and function, understands how

these may be similar or different across diverse ethnicities, gains experience in how these ranges of qualities can be manipulated, and appreciates how each patient's cultural perspective informs their aesthetic goals.

The worldwide cosmetic surgery market is estimated to have risen 57% between 2016 and 2022, and not all of this growth has occurred in North America. This issue of *Facial Plastic Surgery Clinics of North America* shares the knowledge, perspectives, experience, and expertise of globally renowned surgeons. As we move closer together, understanding, appreciating, and respecting different paradigms of beauty can bring us closer together for the benefit of our patients.

Anthony P. Sclafani, MD, MBA, FACS
Department of Otolaryngology- Head & Neck
Surgery, Weill Cornell Medicine, 1305 York
Avenue, Suite Y-5, Weill Greenberg Center, New
York, NY 10021, USA

E-mail address:
ans9243@med.cornell.edu

Facial Plast Surg Clin N Am 30 (2022) ix
https://doi.org/10.1016/j.fsc.2022.09.001
1064-7406/22/© 2022 Published by Elsevier Inc.

Preface
Facial Plastic Surgery: A global specialty that encompasses all ethnic groups

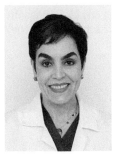

Roxana Cobo, MD

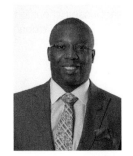

Anthony E. Brissett, MD, FACS

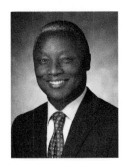

Kofi Boahene, MD

Editors

The editors of this issue are honored to offer an issue that focuses on facial plastic surgery strategies and techniques emphasizing the care of patients of varying races and ethnicities.

Beauty is an ever-changing concept, a concept that has been influenced over the years by the different methods used by civilizations to transmit information. Today, cultures have merged, and concepts of beauty do not have frontiers or races. Over the past several decades, we have experienced a cultural shift globally; as a society, we have embraced more universal concepts of beauty and the uniqueness of racial and ethnic facial characteristics. Furthermore, our specialty has enjoyed a dramatic increase in patients of various races and ethnicities choosing to explore options for facial plastic surgery. In addition to these changes, we are also experiencing patients increasingly expressing a desire for outcomes that emphasize racial and cultural preservation.

Against this background, cultural competency and cultural awareness are increasingly becoming a sine qua non of progressive professional organizations; medicine is no different. This issue is a reflection of our specialty's cognizance and desire to promote awareness and mastery as it relates to culturally sensitive facial plastic surgery practices.

In this issue, we offer our readers a wide range of cosmetic procedures that are performed in our specialty with a focus on race, culture, and ethnicity. This is an issue that covers topics that are common procedures globally. For the readers, we are encouraged to present you with different techniques, points of view, and approaches. As experts in the area of facial plastic surgery, we are committed to trying to reach a midpoint between what is posted in social media with all its illusions and what we in reality can achieve as surgeons. A real challenge, but one that we as specialists should be capable of solving. We would like to thank all the authors that have contributed their expertise to this issue.

Roxana Cobo, MD
Private Practice
Department of Otolaryngology
Carrera 38A #5A-100
Consultorio 222A
Clinica Imbanaco
Cali, Colombia

Facial Plast Surg Clin N Am 30 (2022) xi–xii
https://doi.org/10.1016/j.fsc.2022.08.012
1064-7406/22/© 2022 Published by Elsevier Inc.

Anthony E. Brissett, MD, FACS
Department of Otolarynoglogy–
Head and Neck Surgery
Division of Facial Plastic and Reconstructive
Surgery
Houston Methodist Hospital
Weill Cornell College of Medicine
6500 Fannis Street, Suite 1701
Houston, TX 77030, USA

Kofi Boahene, MD
Division of Facial Plastic and Reconstructive
Surgery
The Johns Hopkins School of Medicine
The Johns Hopkins Facial Plastic and
Reconstructive Surgery center
10803 falls Road, Suite 2500
Lutherville, MD 21093, USA

E-mail addresses:
rcobo@imbanaco.com.co (R. Cobo)
aebrissett@houstonmethodist.org (A.E. Brissett)
dboahen1@jhmi.edu (K. Boahene)

Global Perspectives on Beauty

Blake S. Raggio, MD[a],*, Peter A. Adamson, OOnt, MD, FRCSC, FACS[b,1]

KEYWORDS

• Global • Beauty • Biology • Evolution • Multicultural • Cosmetic • Surgery

KEY POINTS

• Beauty, a powerful and existential force that impacts everyone, can be described philosophically, quantified mathematically, and defined biologically.
• What each person perceives as "natural" beauty is not only genetically derived but also influenced by their demographic environment and artificial beauty as accepted within their culture.
• Standards of attractiveness and beauty are perceived similarly among all humans, but different races, cultures, and ethnicities demonstrate many unique characteristics.
• The evolution of standards of attractiveness and beauty is accelerating due to globalization, with factors such as immigration, social media, and even the pandemic playing influential roles.
• Our individual and societal global perspectives on beauty may be influenced in the future by neuro-psychiatric and biopsychological interventions.

INTRODUCTION

What is beauty? Such a simple question. A question that has captured the attention of the greatest philosophers, mathematicians, biologists, scholars, artists, writers, and dreamers of all ages. An existential and enigmatic question that remains unanswered completely to this day.

As we search for an answer, we know it is multifactorial, evolving, and elusive. We know it holds its unique answers within the perspectives of individuals, races, cultures, and societies. We recognize beauty as a powerful force in our objective universe and subjective consciousness. Beauty is a force that is integral to our human evolution and has frequently altered the course of history. Beauty therefore commands the intellectual scrutiny and psychological contemplation of the inquisitive mind seeking to somehow capture its magical essence.

The exploration of the nature of beauty is especially critical for us as facial plastic and reconstructive surgeons to better understand our own and our patients' perspectives. We must analytically assess individual beauty while appreciating racial and cultural ideals. We must then appropriately use our specialty's tools and our own technical skills to create an esthetic or reconstructive result that satisfies our patients and improves their quality of life. With such interventions, we assume the privilege and accept the responsibility of literally defining contemporary beauty and participating in the evolution of beauty.

With the flattening of the world's perceptions through electronic communication, especially social media, standards are evolving ever more rapidly not only in the major centers but also in the smallest and remotest regions of our globe. Let us begin our journey of exploration and discovery.

TRADITIONAL PERSPECTIVES ON BEAUTY
Philosophical Perspectives

One of the earliest contributors describing beauty was the Greek female lyrical poet, Sappho, who

[a] Alabama Plastic and Reconstructive Surgery, Jackson Hospital and Clinics, Montgomery, AL, USA; [b] Division of Facial Plastic and Reconstructive Surgery, Department of Otolaryngology-Head and Neck Surgery, University of Toronto, Toronto, Ontario, Canada
[1] Present address: 170 Blythwood Road, Toronto, ON, Canada M4N 1A4.
* Corresponding author. 128 Mitylene Park Ln, Montgomery, AL 36117.
E-mail address: blakeraggio@Gmail.com

Facial Plast Surg Clin N Am 30 (2022) 433–448
https://doi.org/10.1016/j.fsc.2022.07.001

circa the sixth century BC stated, "What is beautiful is good." The subject of beauty also captured the attention of the earliest Greek philosophers circa fourth century BC. Plato described Beauty, Truth, and Goodness as the 3 most significant values in his philosophic system. He did say that the good and true were always beautiful, but that what was beautiful may not always be good or true. Plato's student, Aristotle, opined, "Beauty is a greater recommendation than any letter of introduction."[1]

Confucius in the sixth century BC felt the unity of beauty and goodness was simply the unity of form and content, namely, beauty. He felt the beauty of the universe lay in its stability, harmony, longevity, and order.[2] Some Hindus believe that beauty is not in the quality of an object or a person, rather it is in our acceptance of that object or person.

In 1625, Sir Francis Bacon stated, "Beauty is harmony," but followed this with, "There is no excellent beauty that has not some strangeness in the proportion."[3] Perhaps Bacon was the first to know that beauty can be distinguished from attractiveness.

The German Nobel laureate, Thomas Mann (1896–1954) wrote, "Beauty alone is the only form of the spiritual we can receive through the senses." In a simpler thought, Aaron Spelling, the late Hollywood producer, stated, "I can't define it, but when it walks in the room I know it."[4] A more literary English definition from the Oxford dictionary states, "...excelling in grace or form, charm of coloring, qualities which delight the eye and call forth that admiration of the human face and figure or other objects."[5]

It is seen that philosophers, poets, and scholars from all cultures since time immemorial have been drawn to explore the essence of beauty.

Mathematical Perspectives on Beauty

Associated with philosophic attempts to define beauty, more objective assessments were being made and algorithms created to unlock beauty's mysteries. Perhaps the first was the Fibonacci sequence (F_n) described in 1202, wherein each number in a sequence equals the sum of the 2 preceding numbers (eg, 1, 2, 3, 5, 8, 13,...). This sequence was derived from Hindu-Arabic arithmetic, noting its presence throughout the world, such as in the sequence of petals in many flowers. Later, it was further noted that subsequent numbers in the sequence compared with their previous number in the sequence increasingly approached the phi ratio of 1:1.618. This "Golden Ratio" has been called the Divine Ratio and "The Most Beautiful Number in the Universe"; it is thought to represent perfect harmony and is seen in measurements throughout nature.[6]

The phi ratio itself was not described until 1597 by Mästlin. Interestingly, it is found in the DNA of all species and is the only mathematical configuration that can duplicate itself ad infinitum without variance. Think reproduction. Does it, therefore, represent a genetically encoded instinctive pattern in our brain? Is this what guides humans to recognize our own species when compared with others, and to innately appreciate beautiful images? If so, beauty may, indeed, be mathematical and quantifiable.[7]

More recently, in 2001 Marquardt[1] described the Golden Decagon Mask he created using computer imaging to analyze the components of faces through time (**Fig. 1**). He applied the phi ratio to all of the mask's component lines, claiming that beauty is universal and that beautiful faces conform to these shapes and proportions. However, some research questions the applicability of the mask to nonwhite people.[8] Subsequent Indian studies demonstrated that various accommodations would need to be made to the mask to reflect beautiful faces of non-Caucasian cultures.[9] Another study placed the Golden Decagon Mask on contemporary beauties and determined that supermodel Bella Hadid was 94.35% "accurate" to this mathematical model of perfection (**Fig. 2**).[10]

The neoclassical cannons idealizing anatomic beauty through facial proportions originated during the Renaissance, but in many ways were dependent on studies of ancient Greek and Roman art.[11] In essence, the canon divides the face into equal vertical fifths, each equal to eye width, and equal horizontal thirds (**Fig. 3**). Anatomic facial features are further proportionally subdivided. However, there are many studies today that challenge the accuracy of these proportions, even as they apply to Caucasian, let alone non-Caucasian faces.[12,13] Fang and colleagues[14] determined that the greatest variability between various ethnicities was found in the forehead height, interocular distance, and nasal width. Nonetheless, some people continue to use these canons as rules of thumb.

Over the centuries, mathematical appreciations of beauty have thus been proffered from all different regions of the world, often incorporating philosophic, artistic, cultural, and religious expression within their algorithms.

The Biology of Beauty

Our innate attempt to comprehend beauty includes a strong biological component, especially when it comes to our face. For each of us, our unique facial appearance expresses our inner spirit to the outer world. Layered upon our passive facial appearance, our 7000 visually distinguishable facial movements dynamically express our

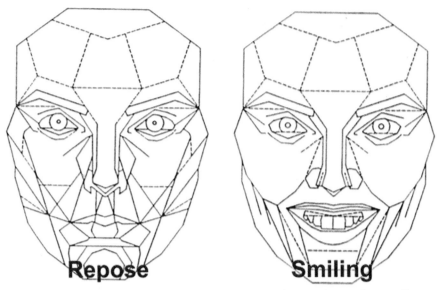

Fig. 1. The Golden Decagon Masks: Marquardt's Golden Decagon Masks in smiling and repose illustrate the application of the phi ratio to each of the component lines; they demonstrate that beauty can be defined mathematically and is a universal construct seen throughout Nature from the beginning of time.

character, personality, and feelings to ourselves and others.[15] For all humans, "Nothing captures our attention like a human face."[7] We all have experienced this immutable, powerful force that can both attract and repel. We have all felt the

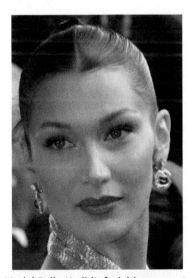

Fig. 2. Model Bella Hadid's facial image matches the Golden Decagon Mask proportions with a 94.35% accuracy, which may make her "the world's most beautiful woman" using this mathematical model. (https://commons.wikimedia.org/wiki/File:Bella_Hadid_Cannes_2018.jpg Bella Hadid Cannes 2018, by Georges Biard. https://commons.wikimedia.org/wiki/File:Bella_Hadid_Cannes_2018.jpg. Creative Commons Attribution-Share Alike 4.0 International license.)

sensory delight and physical response to that which we see, and that which we cannot see, concealed behind the human face.

However, what are the biological and physiologic factors that incite these reactions to beauty? What is really happening when we cast our eye upon another? There are 4 major physical components impacting how we perceive facial attractiveness: averageness, sexual dimorphism, youthfulness, and symmetry.[7] These we perceive in 0.15 seconds when we scan a face.

Averageness or koinophilia

Symons[16] postulates that beauty is a biological construct and has proffered the term "koinophilia" to explain how humans have a love of the average appearance. This concept is derived from Darwinian evolutionary theory that states extreme physical characteristics tend to be bred out of all species' populations, leading to "average" characteristics for the population in a given genetic line. This average appearance is perceived as attractive to potential mates who intuitively know that such a mate potentially increases the chances of their genes being passed on; this is felt to be innate or "hard-wired" into our brains, in contradistinction to being a cultural phenomenon.[17]

An individual's perception of what is average is determined by up to 250,000 images of faces that they have collected and collated from their visual environment to create a composite, most attractive image for them. This process of storing and averaging faces is inherent to all humans

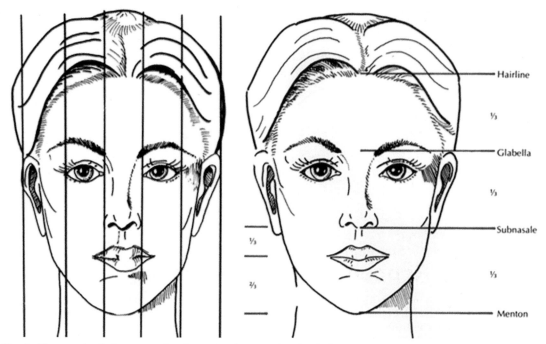

Fig. 3. The neoclassical canons: the Caucasian face can be divided roughly into vertical fifths and horizontal thirds, with numerous subdivisions, to mathematically describe an attractive face; this is not applicable to all races but is still used as a general rule by many.

across all cultures.[16] It follows that our individual human environments are unique, and that our increasingly multicultural world is impacting our individual concepts of beauty. As we visualize more varied races and ethnicities, not to mention many forms of artificial adornment, our inner composite standard of attractiveness becomes more varied and inclusive. Our global perspective of attractiveness and beauty continues to evolve ever faster.

Sexual Dimorphism
If we are attracted to averageness, then wherein lies beauty? The beautiful face is average in all respects except that it has 1 or 2 idiosyncratic characteristics that are outliers from the normal range.[18] Specific features are those related to secondary sexual characteristics that imply higher estrogen levels in females and testosterone levels in males. These more feminine features include large, widely spaced eyes; high cheekbones; small nose; thin jaw; small chin; and short upper lip. More masculine features include deep-set eyes, heavy brows, larger nose, prominent chins, longer and thinner upper lip, and abundant hair.[18] Such characteristics infer good health and fertility and, therefore, potentially greater reproductive success in mating. The concept is that these more extreme physical characteristics would usually have been bred out, but because they have not been in this

particular individual, this individual must have a greater fertility to have been able to retain and pass on these genes.[19,20] Furthermore, women tend to prefer more masculine-looking males midcycle when they are most fertile, but prefer men with a softer, less masculine, and more caring look when not fertile (**Fig. 4**).[7] In today's world, which is increasingly recognizing the fluidity of gender roles, it is expected we will see more individuals expressing heterogenicity in these features.

Youthfulness
Men generally prefer more youthful women, because their feminine features will be more enhanced due to their higher estrogen levels and implied increased fertility (**Fig. 5**). Unfortunately for women, the aging process creates lower eyebrows, nasal tip ptosis, midface and neck ptosis, and soft tissue atrophy; this makes a woman not only look older but also creates a more masculinized face. Many esthetic interventions are geared to mitigating these signs so that a woman can look not only more youthful but also more feminine. Because men have a longer period of reproductive capacity, women may choose men over a broader age range when selecting a mate.

Symmetry
Symmetry has been determined to be a sign of developmental stability and is therefore found to

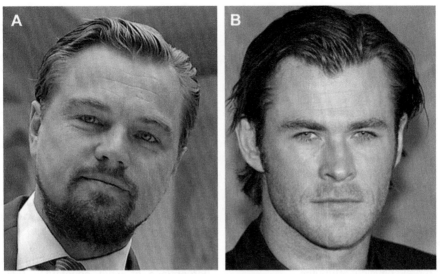

Fig. 4. Attractive male characteristics: Men such as Leonardo DiCaprio (*A*), who demonstrate a softer, more caring appearance, are generally found more attractive by women who are not in their fertile phase. Men such as Chris Hemsworth (*B*), who have a more androgenic appearance, are generally found more attractive by females when they are in their fertile phase. ([*A*] https://commons.wikimedia.org/wiki/File:Leonardo_DiCaprio_2017. jpgLeonardo DiCaprio 2017, by Presidencia de la República Mexicana. https://commons.wikimedia.org/wiki/File:-Leonardo_DiCaprio_2017.jpg. Creative Commons Attribution 2.0 Generic license. [*B*] https://commons.wikimedia. org/wiki/File:Chris_Hemsworth_Thor_2_cropped.pngChris Hemsworth Thor 2, by Benjamin Ellis. https://commons.wikimedia.org/wiki/File:Chris_Hemsworth_Thor_2_cropped.png. Creative Commons Attribution-Share Alike 2.0 Generic license.)

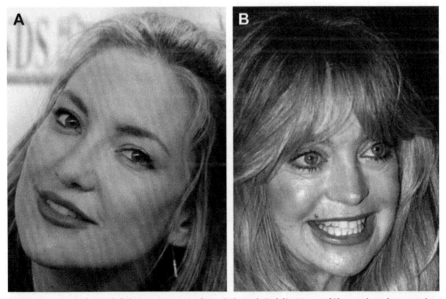

Fig. 5. The attractiveness of youthfulness: Kate Hudson (*A*) and Goldie Hawn (*B*) are daughter and mother. Both are considered attractive celebrities, although neoteny provides an advantage for those seeking mates. ([*A*] : https://commons.wikimedia.org/wiki/File:Kate_Hudson_(25134454051)_(cropped).jpgKate Hudson, by Greg2600. https://commons.wikimedia.org/wiki/File:Kate_Hudson_(25134454051)_(cropped).jpg. Creative Commons Attribution-Share Alike 2.0 Generic license. [*B*] https://commons.wikimedia.org/wiki/File:Goldie_Hawn_(46604499774). jpg Goldie Hawn, by John Mathew Smith. https://commons.wikimedia.org/wiki/File:Goldie_Hawn_(46604499774). jpg. Creative Commons Attribution-Share Alike 2.0 Generic license.)

be more attractive.[21] In men, a symmetric body correlates to an increased sperm count, and in women, breast symmetry correlates with increased fertility. In fact, only about 15% of faces have a high degree of symmetry, which provides these individuals an advantage in the biological sweepstakes, because it is a signal of sexual health.[22] This is notwithstanding a symmetric face alone does not imbue beauty (**Fig. 6**).

It appears that the major physical factors of attractiveness and beauty can be prioritized as to their importance, beginning with averageness or koinophilia, followed by sexual dimorphism, youthfulness or neoteny, and symmetry.[7] It must be stressed that numerous other factors play a major role in the attractiveness of any given individual; these include intelligence, character, personality, and facial expression, among many others, not merely physical attributes.

CONTEMPORARY PERSPECTIVES ON BEAUTY
The Multicultural World Challenges Traditional Concepts

It is recognized that for centuries the study of beauty, at least as represented in literature and art in the Western world, has been based on a narrow demographic. This demographic has primarily been Greco Roman, Western European, and North American. Numerous forces are changing this narrative to recognize the beautiful diversity of the human race and be more inclusive in our analysis and discussions. For example, Coetzee and colleagues[23] reviewed African perceptions of female attractiveness by studying how African perceptions of African female attractiveness are affected by several facial features. The

investigators demonstrated that a youthful appearance, paler skin color, an average degree of facial adiposity (not overweight or underweight), and smooth skin were desirable characteristics. The investigators included all 4 cues in a single analysis, further confirming these were independent predictors of attractiveness. It was also noted that there may be a shift in the African body ideal toward Western ideals. Because these ideals are also favored in European female populations, it is postulated that these may be universal preferences.

A study by Rhee[24] looked at differences between Caucasian and Asian attractive faces. The investigators noted that people want attractive, not average, faces and therefore many of the anthropometric, photogrammetric, and cephalometric data do not really correspond to our general perceptions of what constitutes facial beauty. Mathematical photographic analysis revealed the following for the attractive Asian face when compared with the Caucasian face: facial height relatively greater, middle third slightly longer, vertical "equal fifths" unequal and different, nose relatively wider, palpebral fissures the same, lip thickness similar, lateral profiles similar, nasal length shorter, and nasofrontal angle less. Other studies have shown that the female face corresponds to the phi ratio better than the male; but, even so, the most attractive faces do not correspond exactly.[25–27]

In summary, as much as objective measurements and ratios of facial proportions are similar in defining attractiveness as perceived across all races and genders, they are not exact, and they are evolving across our multicultural world. These studies, among many, demonstrate that

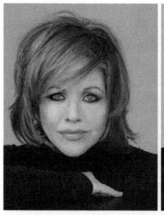
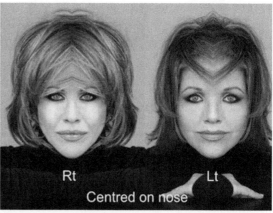

Fig. 6. The attractiveness of symmetry: facial symmetry is attractive because it is a sign of developmental stability and reproductive success. Most people are asymmetric, but many can still be attractive (*left*). Creating perfect symmetry of a person's face through mirror imaging will not necessarily create a more attractive face (*center* and *right*).

consensus can be achieved in rating attractiveness across various ethnicities, genders, and ages. There are differences, but there are similarities, in what all humans find attractive in another's face. Bashour has shown our preferences continue to be primarily driven by our individual, innate, and objective appraisal of averageness, sexual dimorphism, age, and symmetry, rather than our subjective feelings.[11]

Natural Beauty

Natural beauty can be defined as the appearance that is bestowed by one's genetic imprint, and is altered by age, disease, or other involuntary happenstance. Throughout human time, society has bestowed benefits upon those more beautiful; these include better grades in school, presumed higher intelligence, assumed better personality, better service from others, and better pay, among others.[28] Others presume our beauty reflects our inner self—it creates a "halo effect" of goodness about ourselves.[29] Such beauty empowers and provides pleasure. Whether earned or not, fair, or not, beauty has played this powerful role forever in our human lives. Depending on our personal perception, we may feel empowered or weakened by our own personal appearance and how we feel others perceive us.

Natural beauty has also been considered as a holistic concept, one that involves the expression of the inner spirit. To be naturally beautiful, one must believe they are beautiful. A positive body image leads to a strong self-image and enhanced self-esteem, creating a sense of beauty within oneself and an enhanced quality of life.

Dayan and Romero[30] have introduced a novel model entitled, "The special theory of relativity for attractiveness" to define what is needed to achieve real patient satisfaction. The investigators dismiss a "natural" result as being possible following a procedural intervention, claiming it is a misnomer. However, they propose that attractiveness is determined by maximizing the 3 dimensions of beauty, genuineness, and self-esteem to achieve a "natural" result. A fourth dimension is the perspective of the judger.

Artificial Beauty

Artificial beauty is that which is produced by human art or effort rather than originating naturally. Artificial beauty is created to imitate or enhance natural beauty; this is accomplished by emphasizing sexual dimorphism, decreasing apparent age, and improving symmetry. For both men and women, but especially women, this is commonly achieved through cosmetics and fashion; it is less commonly achieved through tattoos, piercings, and medical and surgical interventions. In our developed world, our access to better nutrition and opportunities for physical fitness might also be considered nongenetic ways to enhance our "natural" beauty.

Cosmetic makeup can heighten feminine features such as the eyes, lips, and eyebrows; minimize the nose; and increase a woman's unique feminine signal.[31] Fashion can minimize less attractive and maximize attractive feminine features, as well as make sociocultural and economic statements. Tattoos are increasingly popular in Western societies to express self-identity and cultural, artistic, and personality traits.[32] Notably, in certain cultures such as Pacific Oceana and the Māori of New Zealand, facial tattoos have been a traditional cultural rite for generations. Piercings of all sorts, and ear and lip plugs, can be unique among different races, cultures, and ethnicities (**Fig. 7**).[33] Such devices of "beauty" have been the norm in some cultures for centuries but have increased in incidence in recent years in Western cultures (**Fig. 8**).[32,34,35]

Cosmetic medical interventions such as neuromodulators, facial fillers, varied lasers, and other devices have seen exceptional increases in usage with the exponential growth in these products and technologies over the last generation. Esthetic facial plastic surgery, both for facial contouring through boney manipulation or alterations in soft tissue volume and repositioning, continues to grow in popularity.[36] Of critical importance is that any intervention should provide a genuine, natural-looking appearance; it must appear to be genetic and/or an accepted artifice within that patient's sociocultural milieu. Otherwise, the person is seen as false and not attractive to most others. As any modality of artificial beauty enhancement is increasingly used, it will gradually become accepted as more "natural" and potentially endow more beauty to a person within that sociocultural milieu.

For the facial plastic surgeon, the goal of any intervention is to create a result that appears untreated or unoperated, harmonious with the rest of the face, symmetric, and appropriate to race, gender, and age. Furthermore, it must align with the perceived goals of the patient, being no more and no less; this will improve the patient's body image, self-image, and self-esteem, which improves their quality of life.[37] Furthermore, facial rejuvenation surgery can not only create a perception of youth and increased attractiveness but also creates improved ratings of success and health.[38] With the patient's inner spirit and outer appearance aligned, objective and subjective harmony

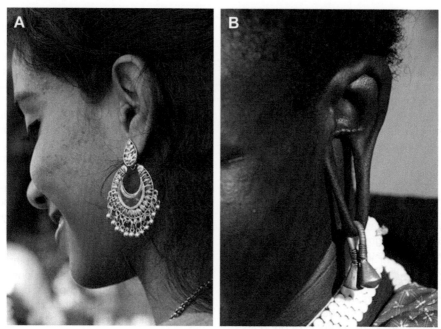

Fig. 7. Artificial beauty: artificial beauty (e.g., earrings) is used to enhance natural beauty; however, such applications of artificial beauty can be unique among different races, cultures, and ethnicities, and is constantly evolving (*A, B*). ([*A*] https://commons.wikimedia.org/wiki/File:Modern_Earrings.jpgModern Earrings, by Isravel Isra99. https://commons.wikimedia.org/wiki/File:Modern_Earrings.jpg. Creative Commons Attribution-Share Alike 4.0 International license. [*B*] https://commons.wikimedia.org/wiki/File:Masai_earring_02.jpgMasai earring, by Hamon jp. https://commons.wikimedia.org/wiki/File:Masai_earring_02.jpg. Creative Commons Attribution-Share Alike 3.0 Unported, 2.5 Generic, 2.0 Generic and 1.0 Generic license)

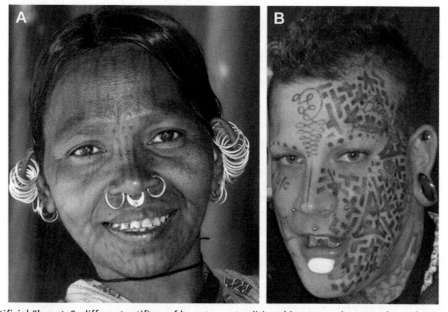

Fig. 8. Artificial "beauty": different artifices of beauty are traditional in some cultures and may be appropriated by others. Piercings of all sorts, and ear and lip plugs, have been the norm in some cultures for centuries (*A*) but have increased in incidence in recent years in Western cultures (*B*). As a new artifice becomes more commonplace, it may be perceived as more attractive in that culture. ([*A*] https://commons.wikimedia.org/wiki/File:Kutia_kondh_woman_3.jpgKutia kondh woman, by PICQ. https://commons.wikimedia.org/wiki/File:Kutia_kondh_woman_3.jpg. Creative Commons Attribution-Share Alike 4.0 International, 3.0 Unported, 2.5 Generic, 2.0 Generic and 1.0 Generic license [*B*] https://commons.wikimedia.org/wiki/File:Face_tattoo_Sevilla.jpgFace tattoo Sevilla, by TUERTO. https://commons.wikimedia.org/wiki/File:Face_tattoo_Sevilla.jpg. Creative Commons Attribution-Share Alike 3.0 Unported license)

are achieved. True natural beauty is realized. As Valéry,[39] the French poet, has opined, "We have a spiritual longing to have an outer representation that matches our dreams, visions and moral aspirations. Our quest for love and acceptance creates our desire for a face and body that others want to look at and know."[39]

Reconstructive Beauty

Most publications presenting studies and opinions on beauty are based on the "normal" face, and not on one that has been deformed by congenital, traumatic, or ablative events that require reconstruction. One study of patients with facial injuries revealed they had an overall level of appearance concerns like those of the general population.[40] Women and younger individuals had a significantly higher appearance concern at baseline levels, and changes in appearance concern were strongly associated with psychological distress. It was concluded that appearance concern is severe among some injured individuals, and that interventions should be directed at cognitive bias and psychological distress. Another study compared esthetic (AG) and reconstructive surgery (RG) groups of patients beside a control group (CG).[41] Each individual completed a Socio-Demographic Questionnaire, Life-Satisfaction Index (LSI), Self-Esteem Inventory (SEI), and Body-Image Inventory (BII). The LSI was similar for all 3 groups, although the RG was the lowest. The AG demonstrated a higher SEI than the RG, which was lower than the CG. BII showed no difference between the 3 groups. The investigators concluded that people seeking esthetic surgery should not be construed as psychologically abnormal as a matter of course but should be evaluated individually. Also, patients seeking further esthetic refinement following reconstructive procedures should be treated as pure esthetic patients.

Ishii and colleagues[42] have studied the social perceptions of facial paralysis. The investigators noted that quality-of-life studies show that such patients suffer from social isolation and stress relating to the perceived negative perception of their deformity. Paralyzed faces were 1 standard deviation less attractive than normal, and whereas attractiveness ratings increased when normals smiled, this did not hold true with paralyzed faces. It is known that facial deformities create an "attentional bias" and distract the observer's attention from the usual eyes and mouth to the deformity itself.[43]

It is a principle of facial reconstruction that form follows function, but it is increasingly recognized by reconstructive facial surgeons that it is also imperative to maximize their patient's normalcy, indeed attractiveness, to achieve their goals and greater acceptance by society.

The Impact of Social Media

Social media and patients

It can be argued it all began in 1965 with Marshall McLuhan's[44] prophetic statement, "The medium is the message," meaning the method used to communicate information has a significant impact on the message being delivered. To that effect, Internet users have more than doubled over the past 10 years with more than 90% of those users engaging in social media, equating to 58.4% of the world's total population. The typical user visits an average of 7.5 different social media platforms each month, averaging 2.5 hours daily or roughly 15% of their waking lives on social media.[45]

Of great importance to esthetic health care providers is the impact that social media, especially shared images and "selfies," are having on our perceptions of our own and others' appearance. This issue has gained greater prominence with the exponential use of Zoom and similar video conferencing platforms because of the coronavirus disease 2019 (COVID-19) pandemic. Patients increasingly have more exposure and interaction on such platforms, with patients looking to social media to frame their personal concept of beauty, identify trends, and interact with other patients and esthetic surgeons. Social media "influencers" are impacting perceptions of idealized beauty.[46]

A recent US Senate hearing on the impact of social media revealed that use of Instagram negatively impacted the body image of 1 in 3 teenagers.[47] These concerning findings may be related, in part, to the recognition that the angle and close distance at which selfies are taken distort spatial dimensions and can lead to appearance dissatisfaction. Software embedded in platforms such as Snapchat and Facetune can solve this concern in seconds, leading to a pleasing, filtered photograph and the desired number of "likes" by "friends." Now each person can establish one's personal standard of beauty for all the world to see. "Snapchat dysmorphia" has patients seeking esthetic surgery to look like their best filtered self, often an unattainable fantasy.[48]

More patients, seeing themselves on video conferencing platforms (eg, Zoom) for protracted periods, are becoming increasingly dissatisfied with their appearance and seeking esthetic interventions.[49] This is despite most users knowing that webcams distort video quality, especially at short distances, where the nose can appear 30% larger and the face more rounded with wider set eyes.[50]

It is indisputable that the global use of social media is impacting our impressions of what we perceive as normal and attractive, not only in ourselves but also in others. What will be the ultimate influence of these phenomena on the evolution of beauty standards for individuals and cultures?

Intuitively, there is an increasing number of people who suffer from simple body part dissatisfaction to body dysmorphic syndrome; this is estimated at 0.7% to 2.4% of the general population but 12% to 15% of all patients undergoing cosmetic surgery.[51–54] All providers of facial esthetic procedures will face increasing challenges to determine what patients want, and whether they will be satisfied with the result. Do they want to look their best in person, in a selfie, or on video conferencing?

An existential question becomes, are we providing interventions to improve one's appearance in real life or through a webcam or selfie? Can we do both? How? Are individuals who wish to look like someone else (eg, a celebrity) pathologic psychologically, or do they represent the "new normal?"

Social media and facial plastic surgeons

Although social media impacts every user differently, patients seeking facial plastic surgery bring their new, often distorted, image of beauty and their often unrealistic, unattainable, and undesirable requests to us to fulfill. It is therefore critical that physicians are knowledgeable about the effects of social media on their patients so they can counsel them wisely; this can be especially challenging, because frequently there are psychological overlays to many of their concerns.

Physicians frequently market their practice through social media. Virtually always they will show their best results, potentially creating unrealistic expectations and increased patient dissatisfaction.[55]

The use of social media by physicians can also create ethical dilemmas.[56] One analysis showed that 63% of posts on Instagram originated from plastic surgeons, with 83% of them being self-promotional.[57] The 4 principles of medical ethics include autonomy, justice, beneficence, and nonmaleficence.[58] These principles can each and all be violated by the plastic surgery influencer who receives or provides payment for promotion. If such information, especially as it pertains to the reality of results and patient expectations, is not accurate, then the patient is open to harm and the physician to unethical behavior.

Of note, 95% of patients review Internet information, with 46% exploring social media specifically, to learn about their procedure of interest. Sixty-three percent use social media platforms as their first search method.[59] This global social media phenomenon is impacting patients' perception of standards of beauty, of what is realistic or not, and what is attainable or not. Patients come to us with more knowledge, although not always accurate, and are more demanding. From the physicians' perspective, we are not only having our own concepts of attractiveness and beauty influenced by social media but also influencing our patients and our colleagues. The rate of evolution of standards of attractiveness and beauty is accelerating rapidly because of social media, with only new platforms and influencers in sigh.

The globalization of beauty

Attractiveness, and its exalted partner, beauty, are first and foremost created through the genetics of reproduction. The ease of travel has increased dramatically in the last century, thus enabling emigration and immigration and a vastly expanded intermixing of the gene pool. This intermixing continues to create more mosaic nations and cultures and is generating greater genetic diversity and more inclusive norms of appearance. In addition, many and varied forms of media increasingly have a global outreach, bombarding everyone in every corner of the world with more and different faces to scan. These multiracial, multicultural faces reflect not only their unique genetic phenotype but also the influence of artificial applications and adornment of self-perceived beauty (**Fig. 9**). Esthetic procedures further alter our standards. Social media is an accelerant to these rapidly evolving changes.

An Allure magazine poll revealed 77% of respondents believe that there is no longer an "all-American" look.[60] Respondents believed that women of mixed race represented the "epitome of beauty." Unpublished research from the London School of Economics opined there would be a progressive increase in multicultural "exotic" physical attributes in addition to sexually dimorphic traits in men and women. A "look to the future" postulated that perhaps attractive faces in the year 3000 would be those of wrestler Dwayne Johnson ("The Rock") and pop star Beyoncé Knowles (**Fig. 10**).[61] Another study felt that our diet would evolve away from meat and that we would develop a smaller lower face and larger cranium.[62] Many rhinoplasty surgeons would concur that the esthetic trend today is more toward a "global" nose—one that is larger, more projected, and has a stronger profile. Interestingly, though, a lighter skin tone is considered to convey luxury and status in some darker races, yet 70% of Caucasian Americans desire a darker skin tone.[63]

According to Poran, "there was once a white norm, a black norm, a Latino norm, and an Asian

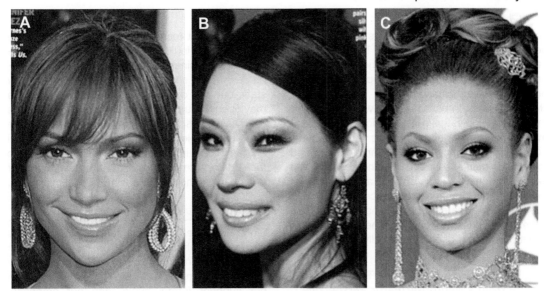

Fig. 9. The globalization of beauty: as individuals around the globe are increasingly exposed to facial images from different races and cultures (*A*, Jennifer Lopez; *B*, Lucy Liu; *C*, Beyonce Knowles), their personal standards of attractiveness are evolving to include those of a different appearance than their own race, culture, and ethnicity. ([*A*] https://commons.wikimedia.org/wiki/File:TIFF_2019_jlo_(1_of_1)_(48696670846)_(cropped).jpgTIFF 2019 jlo, by John Bauld. https://commons.wikimedia.org/wiki/File:TIFF_2019_jlo_(1_of_1)_(48696670846)_(cropped).jpg. Creative Commons Attribution 2.0 Generic license. [*B*] https://commons.wikimedia.org/wiki/File:Lucy_Liu_Cannes_2008.jpgLucy Liu Cannes 2008, by Georges Biard. https://commons.wikimedia.org/wiki/File:Lucy_Liu_Cannes_2008.jpg. Creative Commons Attribution-Share Alike 3.0 Unported license. [*C*] https://commons.wikimedia.org/wiki/File:Beyonc%C3%A9_Army.mil_2.jpgBeyoncé Army.mil, by Jennette F. Everett. https://commons.wikimedia.org/wiki/File:Beyonc%C3%A9_Army.mil_2.jpg. This file is a work of a U.S. Army soldier or employee, taken or made as part of that person's official duties. As a work of the U.S. federal government, it is in the public domain in the United States.)

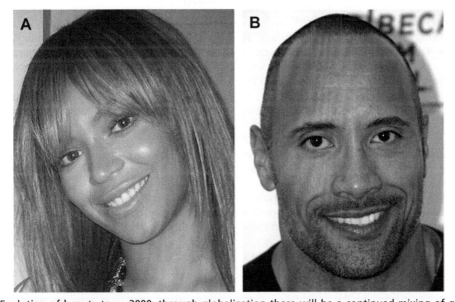

Fig. 10. Evolution of beauty to AD 3000: through globalization there will be a continued mixing of genes and evolving standards of beauty through koinophilia. The average "attractive" appearance in the year AD 3000 could reflect this homogenization of the human race, as depicted by pop-star Beyonce Knowles (*A*) and wrestler Dwayne Johnson (*B*). ([*A*] https://commons.wikimedia.org/wiki/File:Beyonce_in_2008.jpgBeyonce in 2008, by Jennifer-Meg. https://commons.wikimedia.org/wiki/File:Beyonce_in_2008.jpg. Creative Commons Attribution 3.0 Unported license. [*B*] https://commons.wikimedia.org/wiki/File:Dwayne_Johnson_at_the_2009_Tribeca_Film_Festival.jpgDwayne Johnson at the 2009 Tribeca Film Festival, by David Shankbone. https://commons.wikimedia.org/wiki/File:Dwayne_Johnson_at_the_2009_Tribeca_Film_Festival.jpg. This work has been released into the public domain by its author, David Shankbone. This applies worldwide.)

norm, among others."[64] These standards have become increasingly mixed and less distinct in heterogeneous cultures. Over time, this will undoubtedly continue, potentially approaching composite, universal standards of facial beauty. However, in the meantime, it is well recognized that in providing esthetic interventions it is imperative to respect not only a patient's stated esthetic goals but also their cultural and ethnic background to maintain their essence. This mandates all health care providers know what these are, know what their patient seeks, and strive to create an objective result that creates subjective harmony for their patient and, parenthetically, for their culture. This is but one aspect of being culturally sensitive.

THE FUTURE IMPACT OF BEAUTY
Beauty from a Neuropsychiatric Perspective

Just as it was only yesterday that was today's future, tomorrow's impact of beauty and our global perspective is already being felt, and imagined, today. With the rapid evolution of investigative tools, we are learning that being a beautiful person can increase a person's satisfaction with life and happiness.[65] Furthermore, sad people are perceived as less beautiful,[66] and it is easier for an observer to perceive the emotions behind an attractive when compared with a less attractive face.[67] It has been shown that even blind individuals can perceive beauty, implying that our sensory perceptions are not merely visual.[68] We also know, both empirically and through studies, that our minds prefer to view esthetically pleasing people, objects, and scenes when compared with less attractive ones, because this provides us with an intrinsic psychological reward.[69]

Body dysmorphic disorder continues to present a perplexing and challenging condition for facial plastic surgeons, with 71% to 76% of such patients seeking esthetic surgery to correct their perceived deformities, especially their skin, hair, and nose.[70] Surgery is rarely successful and compounds the patient's dissatisfaction, promoting even more surgeries. Studies show the root cause of this defect may be perceptual rather than psychological. If this is, indeed, a problem in visual processing, could the future bring a focused neurosurgical stimulatory intervention that might alleviate this condition?

A contemporary issue is the recognition that facial analysis and identification algorithms do not identify nonwhite faces accurately. It has also been shown that they are universally unable to classify nonbinary genders.[70] Notwithstanding the exceptional advances in machine learning, it is inherent upon us to create facial identification algorithms that recognize the increasing diversity of humans as individuals so as to eliminate algorithmic discrimination. As artificial intelligence becomes more sophisticated analyzing not only static but also dynamic facial parameters, portals may open to diagnose and treat disease processes such as parkinsonism and multiple sclerosis.[70] We may also be able to better assess the psychological and emotional impact of congenital and traumatic facial deformities on a person, and the degree of improvement they achieve with surgical correction.

Beauty from a Biopsychological Perspective

Eighty-three percent of our sensory information is derived from what we see.[70] Our visual perception of beauty is formulated in our occipital gyrus, our esthetic judgment and cognition formulated in our superior frontal gyrus, and our emotional response to visual and auditory input determined in the medial orbitofrontal cortex.[51] Dopamine is released as our neurologic reward for the beautiful encounters that we experience. As the emotions of beauty are known to be realized from neurotransmitters, we might ponder what future biochemical and pharmacologic interventions might be used to treat dysmorphia or even alter our perceived "standards" of attractiveness and beauty.

The Influence of Coronavirus Disease 2019 on Beauty

It is known that an infant's earliest images of its mother play a significant role in the infant developing an esthetic capacity.[71] We might wonder what will be the impact of so many infants and children on their developing standards of facial attractiveness and beauty when they are growing up with masked humans all around them? A Cardiff University study made some interesting, and ironic, findings.[72] Before the pandemic, mask wearers were perceived as less attractive, perhaps because masks were associated with disease or illness. Now, mask wearers are perceived as more attractive than even nonmasked individuals, perhaps because they reflect better health or a caring personality. The most attractive masks were the standard worn by medical personnel, not the various other iterations worn during the pandemic. It is also postulated that this may be because we focus more on the eyes. Furthermore, a visualized hemiface was perceived as more attractive than a full face. Perhaps this confirms symmetry as a sign of reproductive health, as the observing eye fills in the unseen hemiface creating a symmetric and, therefore, more attractive face.

These changes in perception over only a few months strengthen the argument for koinophilia being a major factor in the development of our perception of attractiveness. Consider also for a moment the cultural, religious, and fashion ramifications of these findings. Our response to COVID-19 is streaming and confirming our Darwinian theories of evolutionary psychology in real time.

SUMMARY

Beauty is a powerful force of Nature that has captured and enraptured us forever. Every human being inherently knows what beauty means to them personally, yet its full essence is still elusive to the inquisitions of the greatest minds. Philosophers have offered both insightful and reflex observations, which demonstrate its imprint on every aspect of our lives and the natural world surrounding us. Mathematicians from earliest times to the present have linked fascinating arithmetic and geometric models defining beauty to our very existence and genetic propagation. Although not exactly defining attractiveness and perfect beauty in our multiracial world, they continue to confirm the universal quantifiability and objectivity of beauty in all its natural forms.

The biological imperative of standards of attractiveness being established through the process of koinophilia appears well confirmed and is in concordance with the evolving standards we are observing in our increasingly multiracial and multicultural world. Our fellow humans who have been blessed with higher levels of sex hormones, which have exaggerated their phenotypic sexual dimorphism, are blessed with greater beauty and the many attributes it accords their lives. Symmetry and neoteny remain signs of reproductive health and capacity, adding further allure to those possessing these characteristics.

Today, it is increasingly noted that most studies and expressions of the human form and beauty have had a narrow demographic focus on the Greco Roman, Western European, and New World peoples. This focus is properly changing as we explore and learn about attractiveness and beauty as perceived by the many other races, cultures, and ethnicities in our world. These findings confirm that we all have much more in common than not, that our standards of attractiveness and beauty are appreciated similarly among us, but that there are differences that make us each distinct. Moving forward, it is imperative that these differences, as well as those of gender fluidity, are recognized and appreciated; they must also be incorporated into facial recognition algorithms which can distinguish such diversity if we are to achieve societal equity and inclusion.

A major sociocultural and personality-driven influence on our evolving perceptions of beauty is that of the various forms of artificial beauty; these include cosmetic makeup, hairstyling, fashion, jewelry, tattoos, piercings, and plugs, not to mention esthetic procedures.

Of special importance to facial surgeons is the increased realization that our reconstructive goals must not only address function but also form. It is only by doing so that we can maximize our patient's rehabilitation not only physically but also psychologically, to improve their acceptance by others and their quality of life.

The impact of social media on our patients continues to be dramatic. On the positive side, they have more shared information than ever on which to analyze their appearance and how to seek and select esthetic interventions. On the downside, online distortions of features and unrealistic expectations of what can be achieved are creating psychological disturbances for patients and are posing significant challenges for esthetic care providers. All esthetic care providers must make themselves aware of these revolutionary changes so that they can provide the best medical care professionally and ethically.

Our future perspective on the evolution of beauty standards has already begun. We know that beauty has neuropsychiatric and biopsychological impacts, which are qualitatively measurable. The future may hold surgical and pharmacologic treatments that could alter an individual's perception of self and others. Our current pandemic and the wearing of masks is revealing stimulating and ironic findings. In less than 2 years, mask wearers are now considered more attractive than nonmask wearers. Evolutionary biology as demonstrated by koinophilia is streaming before our eyes.

Throughout human history, beauty has been and will continue to be one of the most mystical and dynamic forces in our world. Our quest to understand and harness the universal force of beauty continues.

CLINICS CARE POINTS

- It is necessary for surgeons to demonstrate both technical skill and astute surgical judgement to achieve consistently good objective surgical results. However, especially in aesthetic facial surgery, even this will only result in a satisfied patient if their personal objective and subjective goals for a changed appearance are also met. Each surgeon must specifically identify these goals for each patient to determine if they are good candidates.

- Aesthetic surgeons must assess each prospective patient for their underlying psychological status. If a patient demonstrates psychological dysfunction of any sort, the surgeon should advise the patient against the procedure, at least until their psychological status is stable and acceptable, or proceed with great caution to mitigate the risk of a dissatisfied patient.

- Notwithstanding societal trends that occur in what procedures patients request, it is advisable to always seek a natural, untreated, unoperated "look" for each patient. This should be in keeping with their racial and cultural characteristics. This reflects genuineness and an attractive, if not beautiful, appearance that will provide the broadest and longest-term benefits for the patient.

- What is considered an attractive or beautiful appearance is rapidly evolving through globalization. The factors driving these changes include intermarriage, multiculturalism, social media, and expression of beauty through individualism, amongst others. Aesthetic surgeons must make themselves aware of these changes, especially as they relate to patients in their practice demographic, if they are to provide the highest standard of care.

- Social media's explosive use is creating distorted image perspectives through the use of selfies and video platforms, including those that modify online appearance. Such patients pose a risk to themselves and their surgeon in achieving a realistic and attainable aesthetic result. These patients must be identified and managed with great care.

- The primary mantra for reconstructive surgery is to restore function. It is increasingly recognized that maximal potential rehabilitation, especially psychological, can only be achieved through realizing the best possible aesthetic outcome. Furthermore, reconstructive patients seeking improved cosmesis should be treated the same as pure aesthetic patients.

- The philosophy, science, art and psychology of appearance and beauty are integral to the practice of aesthetic facial plastic surgery. Study these aspects of our specialty and apply this knowledge as passionately as one would for the acquisition of surgical skills.

DISCLOSURE

The authors have no conflict of interest or financial disclosures to report.

ATTESTATION

We confirm that the rest of the figures used in the article are all original and were not borrowed from other publications.

REFERENCES

1. Marquardt SR. Dr. Stephen R. Marquardt on the Golden Decagon and human facial beauty. Interview by Dr. Gottlieb. J Clin Orthod 2002;36(6):339–47.
2. Fu X, Wang Y. Confucius on the Relationship of Beauty and Goodness. J Aesthet Education 2015; 49(1):68–81.
3. Adamson PA, Zavod MB. Changing perceptions of beauty: a surgeon's perspective. Facial Plast Surg 2006;22(3):188–93.
4. Thomas JR, Dixon TK. A Global Perspective of Beauty in a Multicultural World. JAMA Facial Plast Surg 2016;18(1):7–8.
5. Brown L. The new shorter Oxford English dictionary (thumb Indexed Edition), 2. Oxford: Oxford University Press; 2002.
6. Hwang K, Park CY. The Divine Proportion: Origins and Usage in Plastic Surgery. Plast Reconstr Surg Glob Open 2021;9(2):e3419.
7. Etcoff N. Survival of the Prettiest: the Science of beauty. New York: Random House, Inc.; 1999.
8. Holland E. Marquardt's Phi mask: pitfalls of relying on fashion models and the golden ratio to describe a beautiful face. Aesthet Plast Surg 2008;32(2): 200–8.
9. Veerala G, Gandikota CS, Yadagiri PK, et al. Marquardt's Facial Golden Decagon Mask and Its Fitness with South Indian Facial Traits. J Clin Diagn Res 2016;10(4):ZC49–52.
10. Available at: https://www.geo.tv/latest/251635-bella-hadid-named-the-most-beautiful-woman-in-the-world-by-science. Accessed February 17, 2022.
11. Bashour M. History and current concepts in the analysis of facial attractiveness. Plast Reconstr Surg 2006;118(3):741–56.
12. Farkas Naini FB Leslie G. pioneer of modern craniofacial anthropometry. Arch Facial Plast Surg 2010; 12(3):141–2.
13. Farkas LG, Hreczko TA, Kolar JC, et al. Vertical and horizontal proportions of the face in young adult North American Caucasians: revision of neoclassical canons. Plast Reconstr Surg 1985;75(3): 328–38.
14. Fang F, Clapham PJ, Chung KC. A systematic review of interethnic variability in facial dimensions. Plast Reconstr Surg 2011;127(2):874–81.
15. Adamson P. Fabulous faces. Toronto, Ontario: Oslerwood Enterprises; 2011.
16. Symons D. The evolution of human Sexuality. Oxford (UK): Oxford University Press; 1979.

17. Penton-Voak IS, Perrett DI. Consistency and individual differences in facial attractiveness judgements: an evolutionary perspective. Soc Res (New York) 2000;67:219–44.

18. Perrett DIMK, May KA, Yoshikawa S. Facial shape and judgements of female attractiveness. Nature 1994;368(6468):239–42.

19. Penton-Voak IS, Little AC, Jones BC, et al. Female condition influences preferences for sexual dimorphism in faces of male humans (Homo sapiens). J Comp Psychol 2003;117(3):264–71.

20. Rhodes G. The evolutionary psychology of facial beauty. Annu Rev Psychol 2006;57: 199–226.

21. Perrett DI, Burt DM, Penton-Voak IS, et al. Symmetry and human facial attractiveness: averageness, symmetry and parasite resistance. Evol Hum Behav 1999;20:295–307.

22. Łopaciuk A, Łoboda M. Global beauty Industry trends in the 21st century. Zadar, Croatia: ToKnow-Press; 2013. p. 1079–87.

23. Coetzee V, Faerber SJ, Greeff JM, et al. African perceptions of female attractiveness. PLoS One 2012; 7(10):e48116.

24. Rhee SC. Differences between Caucasian and Asian attractive faces. Skin Res Technol 2018; 24(1):73–9.

25. Pallett P, Link S, Lee K. New "golden" ratios for facial beauty. Vis Res 2010;50:149–54.

26. Bashour M. An objective system for measuring facial attractiveness. Plast Reconstr Surg 2006;118(3): 757–74.

27. Schmid K, Marx D, Samal A. Computation of a face attractiveness index based on neoclassical canons, symmetry, and golden ratios. Pattern Recogn 2008; 41:2710–7.

28. Clifford M M, Walster E. Research note: the effect of physical attractiveness on teacher expectations. Sociol Educ 1973;46(2):248–58.

29. Thorndike EL. A constant error in psychological ratings. J Appl Psychol 1920;4(1):25–9.

30. Dayan S, Romero DH. Introducing a novel model: The special theory of relativity for attractiveness to define a natural and pleasing outcome following cosmetic treatments. J Cosmet Dermatol 2018; 17(5):925–30.

31. London B. Giving pink, purple and orange the kiss off: red revealed as the sexiest lipstick colour. Mail Online (UK). 2013. Available at: http://www.dailymail.co.uk/femail/article-2397116/Red-revealed-sexiest-lipstick-colour.html. Accessed February 17, 2022.

32. Wohlrab S, Stahl J, Kappeler PM. Modifying the body: motivations for getting tattooed and pierced. Body Image 2007;4(1):87–95.

33. Tattoo M. The Definitive Guide to Ta Moko. Available at: https://www.zealandtattoo.co.nz/tattoo-styles/maori-tattoo/. Accessed February 23, 2022.

34. Body Piercing Statistics. Available at: http://www.statisticbrain.com/body-piercing-statistics/. Accessed January 15, 2014.

35. McClatchey C. Ear stretching: Why is lobe 'gauging' growing in popularity? BBC News Magazine. 2011. Available at: http://www.bbc.co.uk/news/magazine-15771237. Accessed January 15, 2014.

36. New Plastic Surgery Report Shows Growing Interest in Aesthetic Procedures Amid Pandemic. Available at: https://www.allure.com/story/american-society-plastic-surgeons-2020-trend-report#:~:text=To%20his%20point%3A%20Nearly%207,same%20day%2C%20according%20to%20Matarasso. Accessed February 18, 2022.

37. Chauhan N, Warner J, Adamson PA. Adolescent rhinoplasty: challenges and psychosocial and clinical outcomes. Aesthet Plast Surg 2010;34(4):510–6.

38. Bater KL, Ishii LE, Papel ID, et al. Association Between Facial Rejuvenation and Observer Ratings of Youth, Attractiveness, Success, and Health. JAMA Facial Plast Surg 2017;19(5):360–7.

39. Valéry P. Some simple reflections on the body. In: Feher M, Naddaff R, Tazi N, editors. Zone 4: Fragments for a history of the human body—Part 2. New York: Zone; 1989. p. 395–405.

40. Rahtz E, Bhui K, Hutchison I, et al. Are facial injuries really different? An observational cohort study comparing appearance concern and psychological distress in facial trauma and non-facial trauma patients. J Plast Reconstr Aesthet Surg 2018;71(1): 62–71.

41. Ozgür F, Tuncali D, Güler Gürsu K. Life satisfaction, self-esteem, and body image: a psychosocial evaluation of aesthetic and reconstructive surgery candidates. Aesthet Plast Surg 1998;22(6):412–9.

42. Ishii L, Dey J, Boahene KD, et al. The social distraction of facial paralysis: Objective measurement of social attention using eye-tracking. Laryngoscope 2016;126(2):334–9.

43. Ishii L, Carey J, Byrne P, et al. Measuring attentional bias to peripheral facial deformities. Laryngoscope 2009;119(3):459–65.

44. McLuhan Marshall. Understanding media: the Extensions of man. NY: Mentor; 1965.

45. Global Social Media Stats. Available at: https://datareportal.com/social-media-users. Accessed February 18, 2022.

46. Eggerstedt M, Rhee J, Urban MJ, et al. Beauty is in the eye of the follower: Facial aesthetics in the age of social media. Am J Otolaryngol 2020;41(6):102643.

47. Instagram Head Testifies Before Congress. 2021. Available at: https://www.cnn.com/business/live-news/instagram-adam-mosseri-congress-teens-12-08-21/index.html. Accessed February 18, 2022.

48. Rajanala S, Maymone MBC, Vashi NA. Selfies-Living in the Era of Filtered Photographs. JAMA Facial Plast Surg 2018;20(6):443–4.

49. Rice SM, Graber E, Kourosh AS. A Pandemic of Dysmorphia: "Zooming" into the Perception of Our Appearance. Facial Plast Surg Aesthet Med 2020;22(6):401–2.

50. Třebický V, Fialová J, Kleisner K, et al. Focal Length Affects Depicted Shape and Perception of Facial Images. PLoS One 2016;11(2):e0149313.

51. Sisti A, Aryan N, Sadeghi P. What is Beauty? Aesthet Plast Surg 2021;45(5):2163–76.

52. Buhlmann U, Teachman BA, Naumann E, et al. The meaning of beauty: implicit and explicit self-esteem and attractiveness beliefs in body dysmorphic disorder. J Anxiety Disord 2009;23(5):694–702.

53. Kuhn H, Cunha PR, Matthews NH, et al. Body dysmorphic disorder in the cosmetic practice. G Ital Dermatol Venereol 2018;153(4):506–15.

54. Vashi NA. Obsession with perfection: Body dysmorphia. Clin Dermatol 2016;34(6):788–91.

55. Nayak LM, Linkov G. Social Media Marketing in Facial Plastic Surgery: What Has Worked? Facial Plast Surg Clin North Am 2019;27(3):373–7.

56. Gupta N, Dorfman R, Saadat S, et al. The Plastic Surgery Social Media Influencer: Ethical Considerations and a Literature Review. Aesthet Surg J 2020;40(6):691–9.

57. Ben Naftali Y, Duek OS, Rafaeli S, et al. Plastic Surgery Faces the Web: Analysis of the Popular Social Media for Plastic Surgeons. Plast Reconstr Surg Glob Open 2018;6(12):e1958.

58. Gallo L, Baxter C, Murphy J, et al. Ethics in Plastic Surgery: Applying the Four Common Principles to Practice. Plast Reconstr Surg 2018;142(3):813–8.

59. Economides JM, Fan KL, Pittman TA. An Analysis of Plastic Surgeons' Social Media Use and Perceptions. Aesthet Surg J 2019;39(7):794–802.

60. Brosnan M. Survey: 73% of women find curvier bodies more attractive. ABC2 News; 2012. Available at: http://www.abc2news.com/dpp/lifestyle/survey-73-of-women-findcurvier-bodies-more-attractive. Accessed January 18, 2014.

61. Sands NB, Adamson PA. Global facial beauty: approaching a unified aesthetic ideal. Facial Plast Surg 2014;30(2):93–100.

62. Evolution Hasn't Stopped: This is What the Human Face Will Look Like in the Future. 2018. Available at: https://curiosmos.com/evolution-hasnt-stopped-this-is-what-the-human-face-will-look-like-in-the-future/. Accessed February 18, 2022.

63. Frazier C. Dynamic beauty: cultural influences and changing perceptions. Hohonu: J Acad Wri 2006;4(1): 5–7. Available at: https://hilo.hawaii.edu/campuscenter/hohonu/volumes/documents/Vol04x02DynamicBeauty.pdf. Accessed February 18, 2022.

64. Springer S. Can there ever again be an 'all-American' beauty? April 6. 2012. Available at: https://inamerica.blogs.cnn.com/2012/04/06/can-there-ever-again-be-an-all-american-beauty/. Accessed January 18, 2014.

65. Hamermesh DS, Abrevaya J. Beauty is the promise of happiness? Eur Econ Rev 2013;64:351–68.

66. Mueser KT, Grau BW, Sussman S, et al. You're only as pretty as you feel: facial expression as a determinant of physical attractiveness. J Pers Soc Psychol 1984;46(2):9.

67. Lindeberg S, Craig BM, Lipp OV. You look pretty happy: Attractiveness moderates emotion perception, (in eng). Emotion 2019;19(6):1070–80.

68. Dayan SH, Cristel RT, Gandhi ND, et al. Perception of Beauty in the Visually Blind: A Pilot Observational Study. Dermatol Surg 2020;46(10):1317–22.

69. Sarasso P, Ronga I, Kobau P, et al. Beauty in mind: Aesthetic appreciation correlates with perceptual facilitation and attentional amplification. Neuropsychologia 2020;136:107282.

70. The Faces Issue. University of Toronto Magazine 2021;15. Available at: https://uoftmedmagazine.utoronto.ca/2022-winter, 20, 25, 26, 33.

71. Schmidt M. Beauty, ugliness and the sublime. J Anal Psychol 2019;64(1):73–93.

72. Hies O, Lewis MB. Beyond the beauty of occlusion: medical masks increase facial attractiveness more than other face coverings. Cogn Res Princ Implic 2022;7(1):1.

Skin-Tightening Devices (Radiofrequency) in Mixed-Race Patients

Rafael Espinosa Delgado, MD*, Miriam de la Torre Campos, MD

KEYWORDS

- Skin tightening • mixed race patients • post inflammatory hyperpigmentation • Radiofrequency
- non-invasive • facial rejuvenation • Collagen Remodeling • Energy based devices

KEY POINTS

- Mixed raced patients are looking for safe non invasive treatments for facial rejuvenation.
- Skin tightening devices depending on radiofrequency are safe for darker skin patients because it is non ablative and it does not depend on photothermolysis.
- There are different ways to deliver the radiofrequency energy to the skin, in this article we will cover the most widely used so you can learn about them and you can choose which type of device will be best for your patients and your practice.

 Video content accompanies this article at http://www.facialplastic.theclinics.com.

INTRODUCTION

Six years ago, we wrote a book chapter for Roxana Cobo's book (*Ethnic Considerations in Facial Plastic Surgery*, Thieme, 2016) on the same subject, so on this occasion we will try to do an update on what we wrote back then.

According to the US Census Bureau in the last decade from 2010 to 2020, the multiracial population grew up to 276% and the white alone population declined by 8.6%.[1] Therefore, mixed-race patients in our practices have also increased, and this is important to us because darker skin types can be affected by energy devices.[2]

Skin pigment disorders are a common concern among mixed-raced patients and their doctors', especially when using energy-based treatments, safety has is always the main consideration when choosing the right technology for this group of patients.

It has been considered that the gold standard for skin tightening (ST) is the carbon dioxide (CO_2) laser.[2–6] I do believe that CO_2 laser is great for improving overall skin quality (sun damage, sun spots, enlarged pores, and acne scars) but after the swelling goes away there is not much of tightening as with the RF devices, and the risk of post-inflammatory hyperpigmentation is always present.[2]

Today's priority in our patients when choosing an esthetic treatment is to be able to get back to work as soon as possible, so patients are now choosing noninvasive ST procedures that are safe and have minimal to no downtime without any pain,[2,7] over other invasive procedures.

That is why radiofrequency (RF) technology is ideal, it has a high level of safety when it comes to darker skin types, it is non-ablative noninvasive, and it has almost no recovery time, and unlike lasers, RF energy does not depend on selective

Department of Otolaryngology – Facial Plastic Surgery, Hospital San José de Hermosillo, Boulevard Morelos 340 colonia Bachoco, C.P. 83148, Hermosillo, Sonora, México
* Corresponding author.
E-mail address: drrafael1@hotmail.com

Facial Plast Surg Clin N Am 30 (2022) 449–455
https://doi.org/10.1016/j.fsc.2022.07.002

photothermolysis of a chromophore but rather heating of water. Therefore, all skin types may be treated.[2,5–10]

In 2002, RF made its debut in the esthetic industry as an ST technology, and the Food and Drug Administration (FDA) approved the first RF device for facial wrinkle reduction, a monopolar RF device (ThermaCool, Thermage, Solta Medical, Hayward, CA) and in 2006 it got FDA clearance for off face treatment.[5–8] Nowadays, RF is mostly used as a noninvasive procedure to tighten lax skin, circumferential reduction, and cellulite improvement.[9,10]

Understanding Radiofrequency and Its Concepts

Radiofrequency: It is the electric current produced using electromagnetic radiation in the frequency of 3 kHz to 300 MHz.[2,8]

Impedance: It is the resistance offered by a tissue as the RF current flows (as the RF meets resistance it generates heat).[2,5,7]

Types of RF devices: This is how the RF energy is delivered to the patient and they are monopolar, unipolar, bipolar, Multipolar, fractionated, and combined with light energy sources, vacuum,[2,5,7,8] and ultrasound waves.

Monopolar radiofrequency

Uses one electrode within the handpiece and a ground pad in contact with the skin. At the same time that the energy is being delivered a cooling spray is applied to the epidermis to protect it from heating. As the dermis heats uniformly, this causes partial collagen denaturation that leads to collagen contraction and thickening. This occurs immediately as the heat is applied. Some additional tightening occurs due to natural inflammatory healing response in the form of neo-collagenesis.[5–8]

The depth of penetration of RF energy is inversely proportional to the frequency; in other words, lower frequencies of RF energy penetrate more deeply.[7]

Monopolar RF devices have a more deeply penetrating effect than unipolar or bipolar devices. The RF can be delivered statically or dynamically, and some are delivered by pulses and some continuously with a constant movement of the handpiece. Discomfort during treatments depends on the duration of the pulse.[2,5–10]

One example of a monopolar device that delivers RF in a static mode with a short 1 to 2 s pulse is the Thermage (Solta Medical)[5–7] and a monopolar device that delivers RF in a continuous pulse with the handpiece in constant movement is the Pelleve (Ellman, Oceanside, NY).[11–13]

Unipolar radiofrequency

It has one electrode with no grounding pad; it emits a large omnidirectional RF field around the electrode in all directions. High-frequency electromagnetic radiation is produced by the device alternating quickly the polarity of the electromagnetic field, producing rotation and oscillation in water molecules, resulting in friction-producing heat.[7,8,14,15] An example of a unipolar device is the Accent Rf (Alma Lasers, Caesarea, Israel).

Bipolar

We have two electrodes in this type of devices; RF travels from a positive to a negative pole between two electrodes built into the handpiece; it is believed that the depth of penetration depends on the distance between the electrodes. Bipolar RF is more comfortable than monopolar RF because it has less penetration, so often these devices are combined with suction built in to the handpiece to get to the deeper layers.[2,7,10,16,17] One example of bipolar RF is the Viora Reaction (Jersey City, NJ).

Multipolar

This is a way of delivering the energy throughout four or more bipolar electrodes in one handpiece to cover a large area of the body, heating faster, reducing the treatment time, and also reducing discomfort, like the Viora Vform handpiece that has four or six poles with integrated suction.

Fractional radiofrequency

In the fractional modality we have two ways of delivering the RF energy: one is through needles and the other is needleless. The first is a variation of the bipolar modality; it is composed of mini bipolar electrodes or bipolar insulated needles, and they can also be combined with a light source device to potentiate its benefits.[5] Examples of bipolar RF are the eMatrix (Syneron/Candela, Wayland, MA), ePrime (Syneron/Candela). In the needleless modality of fractional RF, there is one that uses a roller that has a pyramid shape array of metal pins. When the pins become in contact with the skin, RF sparks flow between the pins and the skin causing microscopic channel wounds. This technology is from the Pixel RF handpiece of the Alma Accent. The other needleless example of fractional RF is the V-FR handpiece from Viora platforms (Viora, Jersey City, NJ); this handpiece has vacuum and cooling, and the array of pins alternate the pattern of delivering the energy to minimize discomfort.

Every year a lot of companies come out with new RF devices and each one of them claiming to be the next breakthrough or the next gold standard in RF technology, and to be fair, they all produce almost the same results. It may be in one or several sessions but they will all get an acceptable result. Some might be better in face ST and some in cellulite or in volumetric reduction. Each device has its strong point and its weak point, mainly because of the depth of penetration, the frequency they work, and the amount of effective heat they produce (in other words the way they deliver the RF energy). It is impossible for us to write about them all, but we are going to review four of them which are the ones we have experience with and they are also three of the most popular ones.

Monopolar radiofrequency (thermage)
Monopolar RF is effective for nonsurgical face tightening; it was the first nonsurgical technique developed for this purpose (book). First cleared by the Food and Drug Administration for treatment of periorbital wrinkles and rhytids in November 2002.[2-6]

It uses a controlled pulse to heat specific zones of the dermis and deeper tissues while using cryogen delivered to the tip membrane to cool the epidermis, preventing heat damage. The monopolar energy is delivered for approximately 1 to 2 s depending on the tip used. A pressure-sensitive tip provides uniform application of the tip to the skin, and the cryogen spray is applied to cool the epidermis, preventing burns, blistering, and pain.[2,5,6,18]

Protocol procedure After cleansing of the skin, a marker path is placed in the treating area, and the return-path is placed in a naked area of the back, arm, or leg. A calibration "shot" is then applied to take treatment parameters.

For every patient, the initial settings are determined based on personal impendence levels and heat sensation. With this information, we decide which tip is optimal for the treatment (for the facial treatment we have two options Facial Tip with 900 "shots" and the Total Tip with 1200 shots). We administer half of the shots to each side of the face.

The RF energy is delivered using a multiple staggered pass technique (circle then square on the treatment grid, providing a 50% overlap on each pulse, in body, a little more in face). Three to four passes are applied over the gridded area and four to six passes are applied to vectors and problem areas until a visible clinical endpoint is achieved, every time pulses are delivered distal to proximal and medial to lateral from forehead to neck (do not treat over the thyroid gland).[2,5,6,9,10]

The treatment tip is kept perpendicular to the skin and generous amount of coupling fluid is applied throughout the procedure to keep the tip in full contact with the skin. The tip has a thermometer and is constantly measuring the temperature of the skin to prevent overheating.

After covering the area, with individual passes, then we start a sweeping technique applying energy through an area of two to three times the size of the tip, following an opposite direction of the aging vectors.

We always leave 20 to 30 shots to re-treat a problem area, and before finishing with the last ones we make cooling passes around the treated area to cool down the skin.

When the 50% is delivered, the system stops, so the patient may drink some water and a picture is taken to compare the treated with the untreated half.

There are few contraindications associated with Thermage treatment. It should not be used on patients who have a pacemaker, during pregnancy, nursing, skin cancer, or lupus.[2,7,8]

For best results, we often combine Thermage with other noninvasive treatments, such as neuromodulators, hyaluronic acid, IPL, and CO_2 laser.[2,19]

Bipolar Radiofrequency (Viora Reaction)
This device offers bipolar RF with or without suction depending on the handpiece. The Viora Reaction emits RF energy at three different frequencies, 2.45 MHz, 1.7 MHz, and 0.8 MHz, and a multimode that combines all three frequencies at the same time, so it penetrates at three different depths so you can target a specific layer of tissue or you can combine all three and deliver energy to a thick layer of tissue.[2,7,16]

When the RF energy is applied, it generates an electromagnetic field causing oscillation of molecules within the tissue. This molecule movement generates heat and that causes two phenomena: the breakdown of collagen cross-links improving elasticity of connective tissue for firmer skin, and gene expression of collagen type I and III, resulting in collagen remodeling and production that goes on for 3 to 5 weeks after treatment.[6,7,10,16]

It has two handpieces that can be used on the face: the ST and the facial contouring (FC). They both have the capability of delivering the three energy RF frequencies and the FC handpiece incorporates vacuum; the suction pulls the skin closer into the applicator so the energy can be delivered deeply to target the fat cells.[16]

Skin-Tightening Protocol Procedure

The ST treatment protocol is performed by using the ST applicator. Cooling gel is applied, set the device in mode 1, start at 52j, and go up from there until we reach a point in which the patient feels the

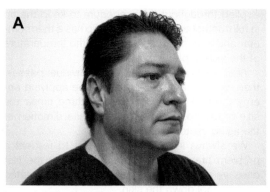
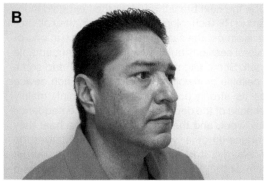

Fig. 1. (*A*) Three quarter view of a male patient before treatment. (*B*) Three quarter view of a Male patient after three sessions of radiofrequency with the viora device with the FC handpiece 3 weeks apart each session, and 3 sessions of the FT handpiece 4 weeks apart along with diet.

skin heating up at a comfortable temperature that should be about 72j. There should be no pain, do two passes on the area to be treated always from central to lateral, and then change into mode two and do four more passes. One or two additional passes may be done in problem areas; you can personalize the treatment to target specific depths just by setting the device on different modes. Several four to six sessions should be performed 3 to 5 weeks apart to complete a treatment protocol and a maintenance session can be done every 3 to 6 months[16] (**Figs. 1–4**).

Facial-Contouring Protocol Procedure

For FC protocol glycerin is used on the area to be treated so the suction handpiece can seal and make effective suction and both electrodes are always in contact with the skin. This is very important because if one electrode fails to make contact a burn will result. Start with one-half of the neck, then go up to the cheek, heat the skin

at a combined mode (mode 4) and a suction level 1 for about 6 min, use an infrared thermometer to make sure the temperature is maintained between 38°C and 42°C, then switch to mode 2 and treat during 2 minutes, and two more minutes in mode 3, repeat the procedure to the other side of the face, and that completes a session, a series of 6 to 8 weekly treatments should be done to complete a protocol.[16] This protocol targets fat cells and loose skin.

Monopolar radiofrequency device Pelleve

The Pelleve is a monopolar RF device in which the energy is applied to de skin by an electrode and a grounding pad receives the energy that goes through the body. The glide-safe handpiece has the characteristic that when it is not in contact with the skin it stops emitting RF to avoid electric sparking and burning; it works by delivering RF energy causing heat that at a superficial temperature of 39°C to 42°C but reaches higher temperatures deep into the dermis and induces collagen

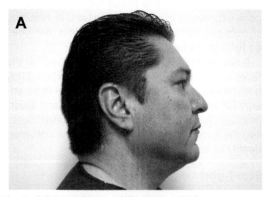
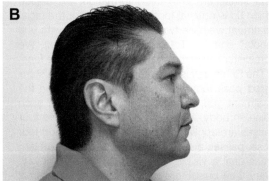

Fig. 2. (*A*) Lateral view of the patient before treatment. (*B*) Three quarter view of the patient after three sessions of radiofrequency with the viora device with the FC handpiece 3 weeks apart each session, and 3 sessions of the FT handpiece 4 weeks apart along with diet, we can see an improvement in the parotid and neck area and a better overall skin tone.

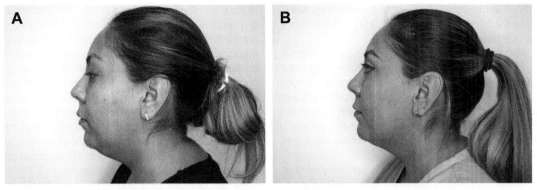

Fig. 3. (*A*) Lateral view of a female patient before treatment. (*B*) Lateral view of the patient after six sessions of radiofrequency with the Alma Accent Xli device with the uniface handpiece 4 weeks apart each session, we can see an improvement especially in the neck area.

remodeling, neo-collagenesis, and elastin uniformity as well. The Pelleve is a very simple to use device, it has several tip sizes, it uses cool gel before each pass, and the electrode is moved in a circular fashion building up heat until it gets to 39 to 42°C and maintaining that temperature for about eight passes, as all the other RF devices it produces skin contraction and contour remodeling as well.[11–13]

Unipolar radiofrequency device Alma Accent

The Alma Accent is a platform that has different handpieces; the UniLarge and UniFace handpieces are unipolar; they have one electrode with no grounding pad; it emits a large omnidirectional RF field around the electrode in all directions. High-frequency electromagnetic radiation is produced by the device alternating quickly the polarity of the electromagnetic field, producing rotation and oscillation in water molecules, resulting in friction which produces heat.[2,7,8,14,15]

This device has a thermometer incorporated into the handpiece for temperature control; the treatment consists in preheating the area and once 40 to 42°C is achieved we maintain the temperature during the treatment for another 7 to 10 min depending on the energy (kJ) you want to deliver on the area; the treatment protocol consists of six to eight sessions 3 to 4 weeks apart, and maintenance once every 3 to 6 months.

Choosing a Patient

The ideal candidate for RF treatment is a patient between 30 and 60 year old, with modest-to-moderate laxity and relatively elastic skin, mild-to-moderate nasolabial and glabellar folds, with realistic expectations, like in all medical procedures patient education and informed consent is a key element in the patient satisfaction.[9,10,20]

Choosing a Device for Your Office

As an advice from my personal experience when choosing a device, take into consideration that the technology you are acquiring suits your needs, requires minimum maintenance, has no or low-

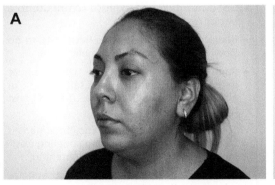
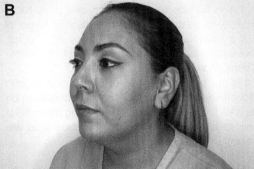

Fig. 4. (*A*) Three quarter view of the female patient before treatment. (*B*) Three quarter view of the patient after six sessions of radiofrequency with the Alma Accent Xli device with the uniface handpiece 4 weeks apart each session, we can see an improvement especially in the neck area and a better tone in the cheek area.

cost consumables, it is easy to use, has well-stablished treatment protocols, and the treatment can be delegated to your staff.

Also is very important to choose a device from a company that specializes in the technology, that has been around for some years, and has a very good post-sale service; most of the big companies would be glad to bring you their device to your office for a demo and have a treatment yourself, which is the best way to decide which device is the best for your practice.

If you are starting your practice, you may want to consider acquiring a platform with multiple technologies; for example, you may have multiple interchangeable handpieces on a single device that offers RF, intense pulse light, nd:yag laser, and fractional RF. This way with a single investment you get different technologies, but on the other hand, if you have a busy practice you may want to have each of those technologies on different devices so you can use them at the same time on different patients.

The most important piece of advice, study your technology, you and your staff need to become an expert on the technology you are about to acquire. This way you can have better results, improve treatment protocols, and educate your patients.

Preventing Complications in Radiofrequency

Complications in RF are rare and often associated with overheating.[6] it is very important to monitor surface temperature during the treatment and keep it below 42°C, temperature below the skin is much higher, it can reach 70 to 75°C. With pulse RF devices avoid pulse stacking because it may lead to overheating and burn. In bipolar RF devices make sure that both of the poles are in full contact, when both poles are not in contact with the skin a sparking burn may occur.[2,8,20]

With the first-generation monopolar devices, subcutaneous atrophy was reported as a result of a high fluence treatment with one pass technique, to avoid this problem a low fluence protocol with a multiple pass technique was introduced, lowering the pain sensation and the risk of complications as well.[2,10]

It is not advised the use of RF in patients with pacemakers, pregnancy, or any skin condition on the area to be treated, and when using monopolar devices avoid use when prosthetic devices are present in the patient.[2,7,8,20]

SUMMARY

Mixed-race patients seeking noninvasive esthetic procedures with minimal to no downtime are increasing; the most common issue in this group of patients when using medical technologies is post-inflammatory hyperpigmentation or hypopigmentation.[3] RF is an energy that is safe for treating all skin types because it does not interact target chromophore; its mechanism of action is the production of heat by shooting electrons into tissue and the interaction with that tissue's impedance or resistance is what produces the heat, and the heat induces collagen remodeling and collagenesis, so skin color, melanin, and hemoglobin do not play any role in RF based treatments.[2,5–10]

All RF devices produce mild-to-moderate results in ST and some devices can mildly reduce the fat under de chin and cheeks; the ideal candidate for RF is a patient around 30 to 60 year old with modest to mild skin laxity. Treatment works better combined with diet and other noninvasive or minimally invasive procedures like botulinum toxin, volume reposition, neck liposuction, especially the devices that have vacuum integrated, and as a post-rhytidectomy touchup.[2,9,10,18,19]

In our experience, understanding RF technology and how your device delivers the energy to the skin and how the energy interacts with the tissue below the skin surface will result in better outcomes.

CLINICS CARE POINTS

- The Ideal candidate for radiofrequency treatment is a patient between 35 to 55 years old who has realistic expectations, with mild skin laxity, mild sagging, who wants to rejuvenate but does not want a surgical procedure.

- Patients above 55 will still get a result, but it will be more discreet because our capacity of creating new collagen and elastin decreases with age.

- Good nutrition and exercise contribute to a better result.

- Radiofrequency treatments have little to no Down time and minimal complications.

- Radiofrequency energy is chromophore independent therefore it is safe to use in all skin types without the risk of post hyperpigmentation.

- The goal of the radiofrequency treatment is to induce new collagen and remodeling existing collagen resulting in skin tightening.

- In conclusion it is a safe procedure that helps rejuvenate the skin by reversing effectively the signs of aging.

DISCLOSURE

Dr R.E. Delgado has no disclosures or conflict of interest, has never been consultant for Solta, Lumenis, Viora, Ellman, Syneron/Candela, Alma Lasers, and is not a stockholder in any of these companies. Dr De La Torre has no disclosures or conflict of interest, has never been a consultant for Solta, Lumenis, Viora, Ellman, Syneron/Candela, Alma Lasers, and is not a stockholder in any of these companies.

REFERENCES

1. Available at: https://www.census.gov/library/stories/2021/08/improved-race-ethnicity-measures-reveal-united-states-population-much-more-multiracial.html.

2. Cobo R. Ethnic considerations in facial plastic surgery. Hershey (PA): Thieme; 2016. p. 372–6.

3. Espinosa R, de la Torre M. Use of fractional laser in mixed-race patients. Facial Plast Surg 2013;29(03):161–6.

4. Trelles MA, Shohat M, Urdiales F. Safe and effective one-session fractional skin resurfacing using a carbon dioxide laser device in super-pulse mode: a clinical and histologic study. Aesth Plast Surg 2011;35:31–42.

5. Atiyeh BA, Dibo SA. Nonsurgical nonablative treatment of aging skin: radiofrequency technologies between aggressive marketing and evidence-based efficacy. Aesth Plast Surg 2009;33:283–94.

6. El-Domyati M, El-Ammawi TS, Medhat W, et al. Radiofrequency facial rejuvenation: Evidence-based effect. J Am Acad Dermatol 2011;64(3):524–35.

7. Beasley KL, Weiss RA. Radiofrequency in cosmetic dermatology. Dermatol Clin 2014;(32):79–90.

8. Lolis MS, Goldberg DJ. Radiofrequency in cosmetic dermatology: A review. Dermatol Surg 2012;38:1765–76.

9. Grimes PE. Aesthetics and cosmetic surgery for darker skin types. Los Angeles (CA): Lippincott Williams & Wilkins; 2008. p. 197–202, 207.

10. Alam M, Bhatia AC, Kundu R, et al. Cosmetic Dermatology for skin of color. Chicago (IL): McGraw-Hill; 2009. p. 87–90.

11. Stampar M. The pelleve procedure: an effective method for facial wrinkle reduction and skin tightening. Facial Plast Surg Clin North Am 2011;19:335–45.

12. Javate RM. Histopathological analysis of tissue before and after pellevé treatment. Ellman Int 2011;1–2.

13. Taub AF, Tucker RD, Palange A. Facial tightening with an advanced 4.0 mhz monopolar radiofrequency device. J Drugs Dermatol 2012;11(11):1288–94.

14. Goldberg DJ, Fazeli A, Berlin AL. Clinical, laboratory, and MRI analysis of cellulite treatment with a unipolar radiofrequency device. Dermatol Surg 2008;34:204–9.

15. Del Pino MA, Rosado Castro RH, Azuela A, et al. Efecto del calentamiento volumétrico controlado con radiofrecuencia en el tejido celular subcutáneo sobre la piel en muslos y glúteos, observado por medio de ultrasonido espacial en tiempo real. Alma lasers 2012;1–10. http://www.accent.com.ar/files/ATT00035.pdf.

16. Paun SD. Non Ablative skin tightening and wrinkle reduction treatment with the reaction system: a three month follow-up study and evaluation. Viora Ltd; 2010. p. 1–2.

17. Adatto MA, Adatto-Neilson RM, Morren G. Reduction in adipose tissue volume using a new high-power radiofrequency technology combined with infrared light and mechanical manipulation for body contouring. Laser Med Sci 2014;29(5):1627–31.

18. Ruiz-Esparza J, Barba Gomez J. The medical face-lift: a noninvasive, nonsurgical approach to tissue tightening in facial skin using nonablative radiofrequency.Derm. Surg 2003;29:325–32.

19. Fedok FG, Carniol PJ. Minimally invasive and office-based procedures in facial plastic surgery. Hershey (PA): Thieme; 2014. p. 147–57.

20. Tosti A, Beer K, Pia de Padova M. Management of complications of cosmetic procedures1-7. Miami (FL): Springer; 2012. p. 23–33.

Hair Restoration in the Ethnic Patient

Jeffrey S. Epstein, MD, FACS[a,b,]*, Gorana Kuka Epstein, MD[a,1],
Abdurrahman "Abdul" Al-Awady, BS[c]

KEYWORDS

- Hair restoration • FUE hair transplantation • Hairline-lowering surgery • Eyebrow restoration
- Beard transplantation

KEY POINTS

- Understanding the ethnic variations in hair and scalp characteristics and the ideals of beauty are very important in managing hair loss with hair restoration.
- Hairline-lowering surgery is particularly effective and indicated in shortening the overly high female hairline in black women.
- Hair restoration surgery whether to treat pattern hair loss or overly high hairlines can be effective in all ethnic groups.
- Hair transplantation to restore overly thin beards or eyebrows can provide esthetic results when attention is paid to achieve flat angulation of hair growth and through the use of primarily 1 and 2 hair grafts.
- The most challenging ethnic groups on whom to perform eyebrow and beard transplantation are those of Asian ethnicity due to the coarseness and straightness of the scalp donor hairs.

INTRODUCTION

It was 8 years ago that I lead authored for the Clinics a similar article, entitled "Ethnic Considerations in Hair Restoration Surgery".[1] At that time I acknowledged the growing number of non-European/nonwhite patients undergoing hair procedures, consistent with the ever-expanding mosaic of ethnicities in North America and Europe that was acknowledged by the other authors in the issue of the Clinics 8 years ago, and is ever more relevant today. This is an evolution every-bit as seen in plastic surgeons' offices as in the Main Streets of cities and towns. Although still "Hispanic-rich," Miami's identity is no longer synonymous with Cubans (who are both white and black Caribbean) but the full spectrum of nearly every ethnic group drawn not only to reside where others vacation but also coming from throughout the world drawn to visit surgeons with strong online presences and reviews that usually reflect excellent work—a phenomenon experienced by my colleagues practicing not only in large cities but also in smaller towns. This global plastic surgery tourism that benefits surgeons committed to excellence is a counter to the similar yet opposite tourism that leads patients to travel to certain recognized plastic surgery destinations where the draw is primarily bottom-shelf low fees. For example, in Turkey, it is estimated that more than $2 billion hair transplantation services are provided annually, an income stream encouraged by a government whose loose regulations of this surgery permit clinics to operate without a physician, rather staffed only by hair technicians.[2,3]

Understanding the ethnic variations in hair and scalp characteristics, various inherent risks of surgery, ideals of beauty, and even the motivations for seeking treatment are as important in treating hair

[a] Philip Frost Department of Dermatology and Cutaneous Surgery, University of Miami Miller School of Medicine; [b] Department of Otolaryngology, University of Miami Miller School of Medicine; [c] University of Miami Miller School of Medicine

[1] Present address. 151 Buttonwood Drive, Key Biscayne, FL, USA.

* Corresponding author. Foundation for Hair Restoration, Sunset Drive, Suite 504, Miami, FL 33143.

E-mail address: jse@drjeffreyepstein.com

Facial Plast Surg Clin N Am 30 (2022) 457–469
https://doi.org/10.1016/j.fsc.2022.07.008

loss as it is in any other esthetic surgery specialty, to assure optimal results, and given our multicultural world, it is not an understatement to say it is critical. It is important right from the start for the surgeon to learn whether the patient is seeking to enhance or at least maintain certain ethnic features (eg, high hairline in east African women, short eyebrows in Asians), or seeking to homogenize with more conventional Western ideals of beauty. In the hair restoration field, significant and continued improvements in techniques and outcomes have provided inclusion as a plastic surgery subspecialty, with equivalent esthetic natural outcomes. In particular, the most significant advances in these techniques and outcomes over the past 8 years since this article was first published has been the enhancement of follicular unit extraction (FUE) harvesting and planting devices that assure higher rates of hair regrowth, the expansion of the supply of available donor hairs using these FUE techniques from the beard in particular and also other body hair, and finally the growth in popularity and improvement in techniques of hairline-lowering surgery (HLS) as an alternative in appropriate patients to hair transplantation to shorten the overly high forehead. Along with these advances in techniques over the past 8 years are 2 advances in medical management of hair loss, first the growing recognition (or maybe the growing incidence) of scarring alopecias frequently imitating androgenic pattern hair loss as well as playing a role in explaining cases of poor hair transplant results, and second the developments in nonsurgical therapies.

Ethnic considerations play a variety of roles in hair restoration surgery. First, esthetic ideals and patient motives reflect cultural norms in those seeking to enhance rather than minimize ethnicity, a trend that has only increased in recent years as people take growing pride in not only individual sexual orientation but also religious and ethnic qualities. Some examples include how Middle Eastern women desire prominent eyebrows or men seek full beards, or how Asian men seek limited beards, or how black men seek flatter hairlines or black women particularly of east African ethnicity are more likely to accept higher but not excessively high hairlines. Similarly, motives for surgery must be understood and culturally respected, for example, how East Indian males (particularly those from the country of India where arranged marriages are expected) will prioritize more youthful fuller hairlines today to obtain a more desirable spouse and disregard the risk of a future of an unaesthetic appearance with further hair loss, or how Middle Eastern men must have a full beard to be viewed as sufficiently masculine.

Important Concepts in Ethnic Differences in Hair Characteristics

The 5 major aspects of human hair
Human hair is generally categorized into 3 major groups based on ethnic origin: Asian, Caucasian, and African. There are 5 major aspects of human hair that vary among each ethnic group. These 5 are mechanical properties, pigmentation, cross-sectional area, curvature, and density. Before discussing these differences, it is helpful to understand the structural components that make up hair and how they differ among the 3 ethnic groups. The hair shaft is mainly made up of keratin materials and consists of 3 layers—the cuticle, cortex, and medulla. In the center lies the medulla, surrounded by the cortex, which is the principal structure of the hair shaft. Outside the cortex lies the cuticle, which functions as a barrier against physical and chemical damage.

Mechanical properties
The hair of the different ethnic groups has different mechanical qualities. Asian hair possesses the most hardness and elastic potential, followed by Caucasian and African, respectively, with damage at the cuticle reducing both characteristics at the hair tip in all 3 hair types.[4,5] When observing the hair of those with African descent, one notes the commonality of hair shaft abnormalities due to the fragility of African hair and disruptive hair styling.[5] Stretching of hair can distort hair structure as well as its properties[5]; this likely explains the greater susceptibility to traction alopecia in black patients. Asian hair has greater stability than Caucasian hair due to its larger diameter.[6,7]

Pigmentation
Dark hair has a high concentration of eumelanin and a low concentration of pheomelanin, whereas the opposite can be seen for blond hair with very little eumelanin and only a trace of pheomelanin. Hair pigmentation is also influenced by the size and density of melanosomes in a hair strand. Thus it is seen that the hair of African descendants has a larger melanosome size and density than the hair of Caucasians and Asians and thus they rarely have lighter hair types.

Cross-sectional area and shape
Among the 3 common human hair types, Asian hair has the largest cross-sectional area and the most circular cross-sectional form.[8] However, between those of East Asian descent we do not see much of a discrepancy between hair thickness. For example, on average, those of Chinese descent had an average hair diameter of 89 μm, Japanese had 86 μm, and Korean had 89 μm.[9]

However, when we compare those of East Asian descent with those of Indian descent, we do start to see some discrepancies with an average hair thickness of 79 μm for hair type of Indian descent.

We also see African and Caucasian hairs having similar cross-sectional areas with 71 and 73 μm, respectively.[9] It is also important to note that the follicle shape determines the appearance of the hair. The typical hair follicle of Asian hair is round, whereas those of whites and Africans are ovoid and elliptical, respectively.[10] The shape of the hair follicle is thus believed to contribute to the appearance and the geometry of the hair. Asian hair has a circular geometry, African hair has an elliptical shape, and hair of whites is of an intermediate shape.[10]

Hair curvature

The curve of hair varies widely among ethnic groups. Asian hair tends to be the straightest, followed by Caucasian hair, followed by African hair, which is more flattened and curly.[11,12] Increased curliness seems to be correlated with a smaller total hair density and a lower rate of growth.[13]

Hair density

An important issue when considering ethnic characteristics in evaluating patients for hair transplantation is the density of hair in the donor site. This density is a product of 2 factors: the concentration of hairs and the size or caliber of each individual hair. The concentration of hairs is presented in the form of follicular units (FUs) per square centimeter; a single FU is the natural-occurring grouping of hairs as they grow in the scalp.[1] A FU consists of 1 to 4 hairs, surrounded by an adventitial sheath, which also contains some supportive structures.[1,14–16] A hair graft typically consists of a single FU, which is the building block of esthetic hair restoration. Asian hair has the largest cross-sectional diameter or caliber, whereas the density of hair is intermediate in whites (whose highest density of hair follicles is 100 FUs/cm^2) and lowest in Africans.[1,5,15] This characteristic may be deceptive to the novice hair transplant surgeon, because African hair gives the appearance of a higher density, given the curly nature of the hair. This characteristic is beneficial to the patient because the appearance of higher density may be achieved with lower graft density in the recipient area. Asians have a high proportion of single hairs (24%–30% compared with 14% found in whites).[1,5,16]

In Asians, the average number of hairs per FU is 1.6 to 1.8, whereas in Caucasians it is 2.3. The number of FUs/cm^2 is as low as 60 to 70 in Asians;

however, as previously mentioned, Asians have a higher-than-average hair diameter.[6,16]

Those of African American, Caribbean South African, and Western African decent actually have the lowest average hair thickness compared with all the ethnicities studied, 71 μm, while still having a slightly higher average hair density than those of Asian descent with 171 hairs/cm^2.[13,16] Those of African descent also on average have a hair density of 50 to 70 FU/cm^2, but because of their curliness, the appearance is very full because it overwhelms the scalp, as touched upon earlier.[17]

Those of European decent, namely, Brazilian, Caucasian American, Caucasian Australian, French, Lebanese, Mexican, Peruvian, Russian, and Spanish, had very similar hair parameters and thus were littered together with the highest average hair density of 215 hairs/cm^2 but without high parameters in hair thickness with 75 μm.[13]

Other characteristics

The Asian scalp has been recognized as having lower laxity than that of Caucasian scalps, allowing the assumption that it could be more difficult to perform HLS,[6,18] which is described later in this article. Also interesting, owing to the high contrast between the dark hair strands and the pale scalp, straight hair, large hair diameter, and the angle of the hairs that grow more perpendicular rather than obliquely out from the scalp, there is a greater degree of transparency and scalp visibility compared with other hair types.

SPECIFIC PROCEDURES
Follicular Unit Extraction

Although follicular unit transplantation (FUT), or the "strip" technique, warrants mention, FUE is the primary procedure used for hair transplantation in nearly all men and a considerable number of women, due to 1 main advantage—avoidance of a linear donor site scar—and several secondary advantages. These advantages are extremely important and warrant review:

- Avoidance of a linear donor site scar, due to how each graft gets extracted one at a time rather than via a "strip." The extent of scarring from FUE, characterized by tiny alopecic "dots," depends on several factors, including the size of the punch, the density of graft extractions (how many grafts are extracted in a single area over 1 or more procedures), how many hairs are left behind unharvested in the donor area, and the uniformity of their distribution and their angulation and curl of growth (eg, Asian hair tends to grow from the scalp in a more perpendicular direction thus increasing the visibility of these circular scars, whereas the curliness of the typical black hair helps to conceal the scars), and finally the color contrast between the dot scars and the native skin (where darker-skinned individuals have an advantage due to the lower chance of having hypopigmented scars).[1,7,9] The development of more advanced FUE harvesting devices like the WAW (DeVroye instruments, Belgium) and the MAMBA (Trivellini Instruments, Paraguay) that use oscillating rather than rotary drill movement and hybrid rather than sharp punches where the "fluted" shape has the sharp edge directed outward allow for improved hair regrowth (due to lower rates of undesirable graft transection of typically 4% vs 10%–15% seen with sharp punches with rotary drills) and less scarring of the donor area due to the ability to use smaller punches typically 0.85 mm in diameter[1,7] (**Fig. 1**).

- Easier recovery, with minimal to no discomfort unlike the first several days of discomfort at the suture line closure of a "strip." The need to completely shave the donor areas (back and sides of the head) for FUE, although still the most common approach used by most surgeons, can be avoided by surgeons who offer the no-shave FUE technique in which the only hairs trimmed are those that are extracted, a time-demanding meticulous process that has as the major advantage no need for any shaving of the head.
- A greater average number of hairs per FU graft, particularly with the first procedure, than seen with FUT[1,7]; this is because with FUE it is possible to preferentially harvest the FUs containing 3 and 4 hairs, unlike with FUT in which whatever grafts are dissected from the "strip," a mix of 1, 2, 3, and 4 hairs, are those with which one has to work.
- Logistically simpler for the hair restoration practitioner, avoiding the need for a large team of hair technicians to do the graft dissection with FUT.
- The ability to harvest grafts from the beard and other body areas. The beard is a particularly valuable donor area, due to the high reliability of hair regrowth and the rapid, typical 24-hour, healing of the donor area.[1,19] As many as 1200 to 2000 grafts can be harvested from the beard staying below the jawline (**Fig. 2**).

There are several disadvantages of FUE versus FUT, which include the following:

- A reduced total number of available lifetime donor hairs, where estimates range from a mean of 6500 to 9000 total grafts available by the performing of 2 to as many as 5 FUT procedures over a lifetime, versus 4800 to 7000 total grafts available by FUE.[20,21] It should be noted that it is possible to combine FUE and FUT techniques, whereby the "strip" is taken from the back of the head and FUE is used to harvest grafts from below the "strip" and from the sides of the head, maximizing the total lifetime number of donor grafts to as high as 10,000 or more.
- The partly erroneous claim that hair regrowth is lower with FUE versus FUT. A landmark study demonstrated outstanding regrowth rates from FUE grafts when harvested by experienced hands using hybrid punches, disproving this claim.[22]

There are indications for performing FUT in the following situations:

- Women who plan to never shave their head, particularly in those undergoing hair transplantation for androgenic hair loss where the density of donor hairs can be significantly highest in the central back of the head from where the donor strip is harvested.
- Men who already have had a prior FUT who recognize they will never be able to shave the head without the linear donor scar being visible, and who request that FUT be repeated, perhaps seeking to combine FUE to increase the total graft supply. However, it is our experience that due to the easier healing course and the perception that FUE is a less-"invasive" procedure, most patients, even those who have a prior FUT donor scar, will choose FUE for additional work.

It must be recognized that FUE is more technically difficult to perform in certain ethnic groups, particularly in black patients, due to the curl of the hairs that extends beneath the skin; this requires special techniques that oftentimes only highly experienced FUE surgical teams can provide, facilitated by the use of the more advanced FUE systems described earlier. Punch diameter needs to be adjusted depending on the size of the FUs being extracted (a factor of hair caliber and the number of hairs per FU) and the ease of graft extraction (sometimes larger punches can facilitate the intact harvesting of certain difficult-to-extract grafts). Certain ethnic groups have typically larger FUs, thus requiring a larger punch of 0.9 mm or even larger.[5,20,23] Because in Asians compared with Caucasians the hair follicles are

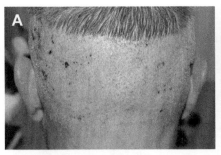
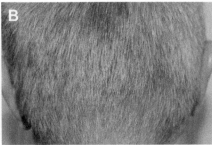
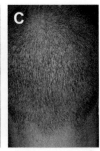

Fig. 1. Patient before (*A*) and 2 weeks after (*B*) FUE procedure, and second patient 1 week after (*C*) FUE procedures.

longer and the dermal papilla that must be cut through to free up the graft extends a bit further from the skin surface, the punch typically must be used to cut a bit deeper.[1,23,24]

Achieving Naturalness and Meeting Esthetic Goals in Patients of Varying Ethnic Groups

An appreciation for the ethnic variation of desired hairline design must be appreciated to satisfy patient goals. At the same time, realistic expectations, with an accounting of future hair loss, must be factored in and shared with the patient in consultation. Listening to the patient's goals and showing of prior results achieved in similar cases by the surgeon can be invaluable. Inevitably, there are 2 main decisions facing the surgeon-patient team— the location and design of the hairline with the tradeoff being a lower more youthful hairline versus a more conservative hairline that will better conserve the precious limited donor supply and the balance of density and feathering of the hairline.

With regard to the design and position of the hairline in males, as referred to earlier in this article, many male East Indian as well as black patients desire lower more youthful flatter/less laterally receded hairlines, the former because of the desire for better marital prospects in the short term and the latter because of ethnic ideals of beauty (**Fig. 3**). Similarly, certain Hispanic populations

such as Mexican and Columbian to my observation have a certain subset of men with quite low hairlines, thus driving concepts of esthetic ideals. Meanwhile in women the ethnic concepts of beauty in this area have in my observation less fluctuation, with nearly all females desiring rounded hairlines with appropriate forehead height that complements the lower two-thirds of the face (**Figs. 4** and **5**).

With regard to density versus a natural appearance, this is largely an individual choice, with some consistent ethnic rules. The appearance of density is due to several factors: the thickness of each hair, the density of hairs (number of FUs times hairs per FU in a given area), the angulation of the hair (more acute angulation provides the appearance of greater density), the curl of the hairs (more curl means the appearance of more density, compensating for the fact that curlier hairs require typically larger recipient sites and cannot be as densely packed), and finally the contrast between skin and hair color with the lesser the contrast the greater the appearance of density (because the scalp is less visible). This lack of color contrast is also associated with a more natural appearance. Other features associated with a more natural appearance are a more acute angulation of the hair, the appropriate application of single and even 2 hair grafts to create a feathered appearance, and esthetic fluctuation of density. In no

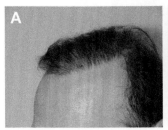
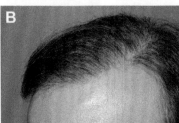
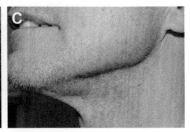

Fig. 2. Patient before (*A*) and 10 months after (*B*) reparative procedure using donor hairs from the beard, which has healed up without any scarring (*C*).

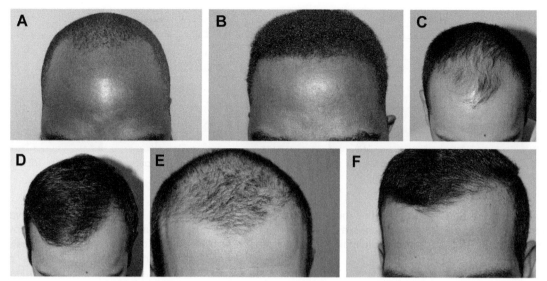

Fig. 3. Black patient before (*A*) and after (*B*) hair transplant with a typical desired "flatter" hairline, compared with Hispanic patient presenting with similar hair loss pattern (*C, E*) and after (*D, F*) hair transplant.

ethnic group is an emphasis on naturalness over density more important than in Asians, due to the high color contrast between scalp and hair, and the typical straightness and large caliber of hairs (**Fig. 6**). Meanwhile, the black patient is typically the easiest on whom to achieve density without compromising naturalness, due to the low color contrast and the curly hairs. In fact, the use of single hairs in black patients is usually unnecessary; instead the hairline can be created with all 2-hair

grafts (**Fig. 7**). Another factor to consider in the black patient is the higher incidence of traction alopecia due to hair styles, as well as particularly in women the higher incidence of scarring alopecias like central centrifugal cicatricial alopecia that can sometimes mimic other types of hair loss, a condition associated with low to minimal hair regrowth.[25] Finally, in typically darker-skinned Middle East and East Indian and certain Hispanic men, the lower color contrast between the skin

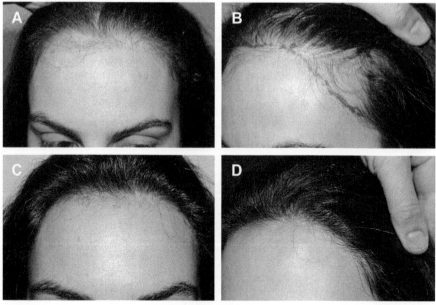

Fig. 4. Before (*A, B*) and after (*C, D*) hair transplant on a female to create the near-universal for all ethnic groups' desired rounded shape.

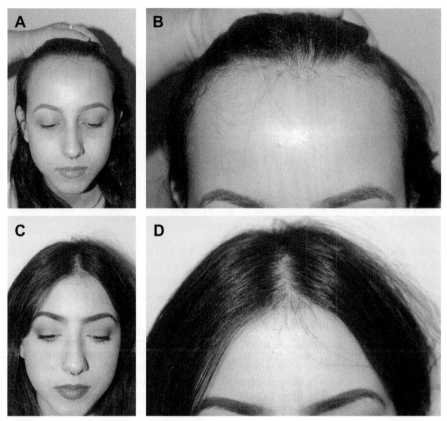

Fig. 5. Before (*A*, *B*) and after (*C*, *D*) hairline-lowering/forehead reduction surgery demonstrating the near-universal ideal female hairline shape and position.

and dark brown or black hairs facilitates the achievement of density and naturalness. This phenomenon mimics the same concept but just the opposite situation as seen in many northern Europeans, where the typically lighter hair color blends in well with the similarly typically more fair skin (**Fig. 8**).

Recipient sites with FUE cases in most Caucasians are made with blades sized 0.5 mm for 1- and some 2-hair grafts, 0.6 mm for some 2- and most 3-hair grafts, and sometimes 0.7-mm blades for some larger 3- and larger-sized grafts especially when there is low compliance of the recipient site skin. Note that in general FUE grafts are around 25% smaller than FUT grafts, reflecting the fact that FUE grafts are often "skinnier" meaning they contain less surrounding supportive tissue than those dissected out under the microscope. These "skinnier" grafts are more prone to desiccation and physical damage during the planting process, a liability that is overcome by the use of graft implanters that facilitate graft placement with minimal to no trauma. Typically recipient sites need to be 0.1 to 0.2 mm larger at each graft size for

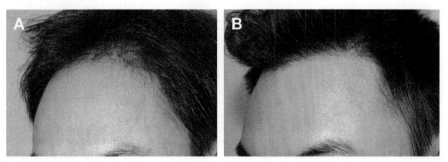

Fig. 6. Before (*A*) and after (*B*) FUE hair transplant on Asian male, where mostly 1- and 2-hair grafts were used.

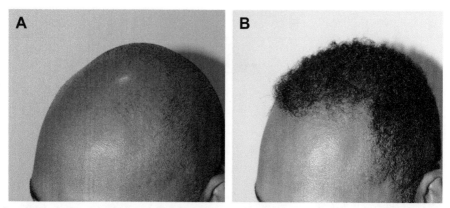

Fig. 7. Before (*A*) and after (*B*) FUE hair transplant on black patient, where even along the hairline 2-hair grafts are used to optimize density without compromising naturalness.

patients of Asian and East Indian ethnicity due to the greater thickness of the FU grafts, and 0.2 to 0.3 mm larger for black patients due to the curl of the hairs. Although typically larger in size (0.7–0.9 mm most commonly), the depth of the recipient sites in black patients is usually less than in other ethnic groups due to the hairs being somewhat shorter.

One final observation must be noted in ethnic variation of graft planting. The East Indian patient's grafts are oftentimes more difficult to plant than in other ethnic groups, due to 2 reasons. First, the darker skin (as in black patients) makes it more difficult to actually visualize the recipient sites due to less contrast between the tiny crust of blood and skin color. Second, for reasons that are still unclear to me, the grafts particularly of Pakistani patients have a tendency to be "oily,"

leading to a greater tendency to "pop" after placement as well as an associated greater challenge of placement into recipient sites; however, the use of implanters significantly reduces this challenge.

Eyebrow Transplantation

The requirements for achieving natural results when transplanting eyebrows are esthetic design with symmetry between the 2 sides, flat angulation of the hairs, the ideal balance of 1- and 2- and sometimes even 3-hair grafts, and proper crosshatching and direction of the hairs. The 2 ethnic groups in whom it is the hardest to achieve natural appearances in eyebrow restoration are Asian and black patients, due to characteristics of the scalp donor hairs (**Fig. 9**). In Asian patients, the typically straight and oftentimes coarse nature of hair

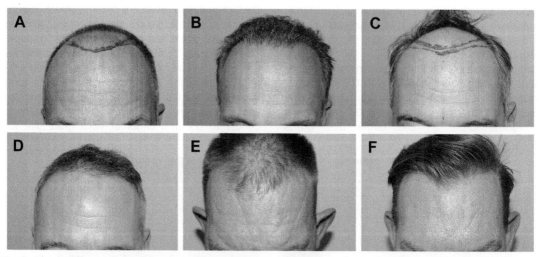

Fig. 8. Three different hair and scalp color combinations of patients who underwent FUE hair transplantation, demonstrating how in a patient with dark skin even when the donor hairs are dark the appearance of density achieved is quite good (*A*: before, *B*: after), in a patient with light skin and medium colored hair the appearance of density achieved is somewhat less (*C*: before, *D*: after), and in patient with light skin and light reddish hair the appearance of density achieved is quite good (*E*: before, *F*: after).

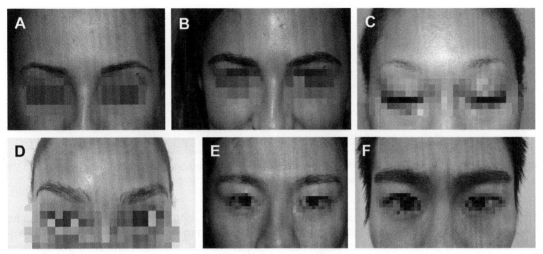

Fig. 9. Three ethnic groups showing result of eyebrow transplantation: Hispanic patient (*A*: before, *B*: after), black patient (*C*: before, *D*: after), and Asian patient (*E*: before, *F*: after).

growth makes it more difficult to achieve flat angulation, because the absence of a curl denies the ability of the hair curling in a direction that complements the angulation of the recipient sites. In black patients who have a "hard" curl to the donor hairs, it can be particularly challenging to achieve uniform direction and angulation of hair growth, resulting in more "rogue" hair growth. To compensate for these challenging hair characteristics when they are present, primarily 1-hair grafts are to be used trading in some of the density in return for greater naturalness. When dissecting the naturally occurring 2- and 3-hair FUE grafts to have more single hair grafts, to ensure viability it is important to leave the single-hair graft with a larger cuff of supporting tissue. These patients are advised that a second procedure can always be performed to increase density if desired. The most impressive results in eyebrow transplantation, due to the characteristics of darker complexion and wavy, reasonably thick donor hairs, are those of Hispanic, East Indian, and Middle Eastern individuals.

Esthetic eyebrow design and size vary among ethnic groups, with certain trends observed. Asian women and men tend to find shorter eyebrows (5–5.5 cm) more ideal, and Middle Eastern men and women prefer thick prominent eyebrows, but these are merely general and not hard rules. One risk we have identified particularly in eyebrows but occurring occasionally in the scalp and the beard is that of black patients developing small bumps at the point where the hair emerges from the skin. Fortunately, this is not frequent, but can occur, and seems to be secondary to some combination of the cuff of skin left on the graft becoming raised during healing, and the relative thickness and strength of the hair pushing outward on the skin. In the few cases where this has occurred, treatment consisting of steroid injections and or superficial skin shaving seems to ameliorate the presence of these bumps.

In nearly all men and most women, the grafts for eyebrow transplantation are harvested using the FUE technique. Recipient sites most commonly are made using a 0.5-mm blade for 1- and 2-hair grafts. In many cases, the 3-hair grafts, used to achieve central density in select cases, are placed into the same sized recipient sites, but if not a 0.6-mm blade is used to make the recipient sites. The key to esthetic results is optimal placement and angulation of the recipient sites, and meticulous implanting—using implanters—of the grafts into these recipient sites, keeping the grafts moist.

Beard Transplantation

No other component of the face exudes masculinity more than a beard, and the desire for fuller beards continues to grow in nearly all men of all ethnicities, age, and working class. Although a procedure requested by those of nearly all ethnicities, the desired beard appearance can vary widely. For Asian men, in whom beards tend to be naturally less prominent and in some cases limited to just a thin mustache and "soul patch" of hair under the lower lip, almost any type of beard enhancement is acceptable. One of the more common patterns desired in the Asian male consists of a relatively narrow strap beard that runs along and extends upward an inch or so above the jawline, well-defined sideburns, a thin

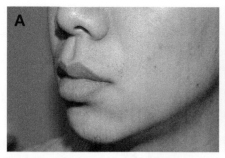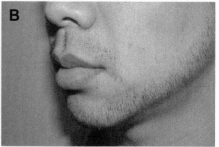

Fig. 10. Before (*A*) and after (*B*) beard transplant on Asian patient, demonstrating the "strap" beard and the outcome when naturalness is best achieved through the use of mostly single-hair grafts.

but present mustache, and narrow but reasonably dense horizontal "soul patch" (**Fig. 10**). Because of the need for using almost exclusively single hair grafts to assure naturalness (and thus compromising density) due to the thick straight donor hairs, such conservative expectations of density are fortuitous, and of all the ethnic groups the performing of a second procedure for greater density is most common in Asians.

East Indian and Middle Eastern men, along with of course the typical Scandinavian/northern European sic Brooklyn "hipster" seem to desire thick beards to enhance masculinity (**Fig. 11**). Hispanic men often have particular desire for a strong mustache, whereas some Hassidic Jews not blessed with a thick beard will seek such for social acceptance in the religious community. Black men can have a wide variety of esthetic ideals for the beard, and because of the increased challenge of working with these curly hairs as well as the small but definite risk of bump formation particularly around the goatee that together dictate for the use of mostly single-hair grafts, achieving density can be challenging particularly in those of lighter complexion (**Fig. 12**).

Like with eyebrow transplantation, acute angulation of recipient sites is required to prevent the hairs from growing at an unaesthetic direction; this is best achieved through the use of the smallest possible recipient sites, most commonly 0.5 mm for single- and sometime 2-hair grafts, where 0.6 mm is sometimes required. It is also important that patients, particularly younger men younger than 30 years, be evaluated for the presence or risk of male pattern baldness, because any hairs transplanted into the beard are hairs not available in the future for transplanting into areas of male pattern hair loss. One way to at least partially deal with this limited supply of donor hairs is to use the beard as donor. Although it can be somewhat more challenging to extract, with experience and the use of certain hybrid FUE punches, beard donor hair has a high and consistent rate of regrowth, and essentially overnight healing without any scarring. When attempting beard hair donation in the black patient (or for that matter, transplantation into the beard), it may be valuable to do a test procedure of less than 100 grafts to assess healing of the donor and recipient areas. A history of folliculitis barbi in the black patient poses a risk of poor healing in both the donor and recipient areas. Hyperpigmentation, although intuitively would seem to be a risk when transplanting patients of ethnic groups of darker or Asian skin, does not seem to be a problem.

The great majority of beard transplants are performed to address genetic thinness, but in certain cases there can be other causes. Prior laser removal, later regretted, can be reversed successfully. The beards of gender reaffirmation—female

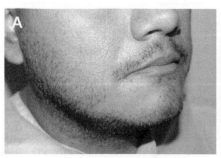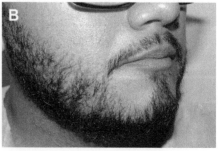

Fig. 11. Before (*A*) and after (*B*) beard transplant in patient of Middle Eastern ethnicity.

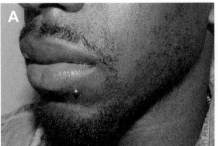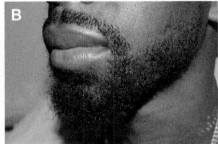

Fig. 12. Before (*A*) and after (*B*) beard transplant in black patient.

to male—patients are limited in the amount of hair growth that can be expected with testosterone administration, and with the restoration of a strong goatee and sideburns, to even a full beard; there can be a nice improvement in a masculine appearance. Other causes for beard transplantation include trauma and previous surgery, and although scars can be more difficult in which to achieve full regrowth, in most cases there can be a nice esthetic result.

Hairline-Lowering/Forehead Reduction Surgery

Over the past 5 years, the popularity of this surgical procedure to lower the overly high hairline has grown tremendously, due to the recognition of the advantages in the appropriate patient. As an alternative to hair grafting, HLS is capable of

shortening the overly high usually female hairline by an inch or more in a single procedure, yielding instantaneous results and unsurpassed density (equivalent to the transplanting of 4000 to as many as 7000 grafts).[1,9,26]

The surgery is performed under general anesthesia, and takes less than 2 hours to perform. After the making of a trichophytic incision along the marked out hairline to assure hair growth through the scar, the scalp is undermined in the subgaleal plane 3 to 6 cm beyond the vertex so that it extends close to por up to the nuchal ridge, maximizing scalp mobility. Mechanical creep (traction) is applied, occasionally a coronal galeotomy made for increased advancement (not usually performed due to the increased risk of shock hair loss), and the now advanced scalp is secured in position (typically 20–25 mm further forward) by paired Endotine clips, whose barbs engage into

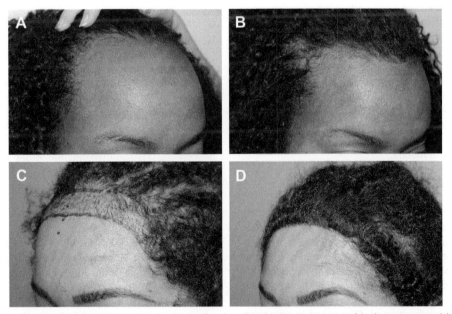

Fig. 13. Before (*A*) and after (*B*) hairline-lowering/forehead reduction surgery in black patient, and before (*C*) and after (*D*) images in another black patient who underwent hairline-lowering/forehead reduction surgery to excise prior transplants and create a fuller more esthetic hairline.

the galea. The excess forehead skin is excised, and the skin closed in a layered fashion, under minimal to no tension due to the engagement of the Endotine clips. Patients are presentable 1 or 2 days after with brushing of the frontal hairs forward to conceal the sutures until they are removed 1 week later. In around 15% to 20% of patients, hair grafting is performed as soon as 3 months later, to conceal any visibility of the hairline scar that can occasionally occur, or to round out the hairline further than that which can be achieved by the surgery.

To be a good candidate for HLS, there must be sufficient laxity of the scalp, and no evidence of thinning of the hairline hairs, otherwise with loss of these hairs the typically fine-line scar with hair growing through it could become exposed with time. Because of this requirement for permanent hairs, few men are safely or appropriately treated with HLS, particularly those aged 45 years and younger. Prior browlift or facelift surgery is usually a contraindication to HLS due to impairment of blood circulation.

The most common ethnic group to undergo HLS are black patients (**Fig. 13**). First, there is a tendency of high foreheads particularly in those of East African (Eritrea, Kenya, Ethiopia, and Sudan) ethnicity, who due to more Western ideals of beauty tend to want to reduce the forehead prominence that is achieved with this surgery. Second, many black patients tend to have good scalp laxity, thus allowing for a greater amount of lowering than seen in other ethnic groups.[27] The concern for keloid or hypertrophic scarring does not seem to be justified in black patients, in whom the great majority have excellent hairline scars with hair growth through it. The desire to correct what is usually a genetically high hairline, which conveys senescence and sometimes masculinity, is not limited to any one ethnic group. Hispanic as well as Middle Eastern and Asian women all frequently choose HLS due to the many advantages over grafting including the impressive, virtually overnight results.

SUMMARY

Hair restoration surgery, whether to the scalp to treat pattern hair loss or high hairlines or a variety of other causes, or to the eyebrows to treat overplucking or thinning due to senescence or disease, or to the beard due to genetics or the undesirable outcome of prior laser hair removal, can all be effective and popular options in those of all ethnic groups. Consideration of differences in hair characteristics, healing, and esthetic ideals must all be factored into the decision-making process.

DISCLOSURE

The authors have nothing to disclose.

REFERENCES

1. Epstein J, Bared A, Kuka G. Ethnic considerations in Hair Restoration Surgery. Facial Plast Surg Clin N Am 2014;22(3):427–37.
2. Behind the Scenes of Turkey's $1B Hair Transplant Industry, by Laura Mallonee, as appeared in WIRED, November 3, 2015.
3. Why Men Everywhere Are Going to Istanbul for Hair Transplants, by Angus Bennette and David Rovella, as appeared in Bloomberg.com, September 27, 2021.
4. Wei G, Bhushan B, Torgerson PM. Nanomechanical characterization of human hair using nanoindentation and SEM. Ultramicroscopy 2005;105(1–4):248–66.
5. Franbourg A, Hallegot P, Baltenneck F, et al. Current research on ethnic hair. J Am Acad Dermatol 2003;48(6 Suppl):S115–9.
6. Richards GM, Oresajo CO, Halder RM. Structure and function of ethnic skin and hair. Dermatol Clin 2003;21(4):595–600.
7. Park JH. A novel concept for determining the direction of implanted hair in hairline correction surgery in East Asian women. Arch Plast Surg 2018;45(3):292–4.
8. Rose PT. The latest innovations in hair transplantation. Facial Plast Surg 2011;27(4):366–77.
9. Coderch L, Oliver MA, Carrer V, et al. External lipid function in ethnic hairs. J Cosmet Dermatol 2019;18(6):1912–20.
10. Cruz CF, Fernandes MM, Gomes AC, et al. Keratins and lipids in ethnic hair. Int J Cosmet Sci 2013;35(3):244–9.
11. Loussouarn G, Lozano I, Panhard S, et al. Diversity in human hair growth, diameter, colour and shape. An in vivo study on young adults from 24 different ethnic groups observed in the five continents. Eur J Dermatol 2016;26(2):144–54.
12. Headington JT. Transverse microscopic anatomy of the human scalp: a basis for a morphometric approach to disorders of the hair follicle. Arch Dermatol 1984;120:449–56.
13. Sperling LC. Hair density in African Americans. Arch Dermatol 1999;135:656–8.
14. Kim JC. Asian hair: A Korean study. In: Pathomvanich D, Imigawa K, editors. Hair restoration surgery in Asians. Tokyo: Springer; 2010. p. 21–2.
15. Ortega-Castillejos DKA, Pathomvanich D. Retrospective Assessment of Follicular Unit Density in Asian Men With Androgenetic Alopecia. Dermatol Surg 2017;43(5):672–83.

16. Porter CE, Dixon F, Khine CC, et al. The behavior of hair from different countries. J Cosmet Sci 2009; 60(2):97–109.

17. Ng Bertram. Idiopathic Occipital Fibrosis: What the Fue Hair Surgeon Should Be Aware Of. Int Soc Hair Restoration Surg 2012;22(6):230–2.

18. Sharma R, Ranjan A. Follicular Unit Extraction (FUE) Hair Transplant: Curves Ahead. J Maxillofac Oral Surg 2019;18(4):509–17.

19. Saxena K, Savant SS. Body to Scalp: Evolving Trends in Body Hair Transplantation. Indian Dermatol Online J 2017;8(3):167–75.

20. Humayun Mohmand M, Ahmad M. Effect of Follicular Unit Extraction on the Donor Area. World J Plast Surg 2018;7(2):193–7.

21. Joshi R, Shokri T, Baker A, et al. Alopecia and techniques in hair restoration: an overview for the cosmetic surgeon. Oral Maxillofac Surg 2019; 23(2):123–31.

22. Devroye J, Epstein J, Josephitis DS, et al. Sharp and hybrid punches: a detailed comparison of different quality control markers. Hair Transplant Forum International Journal 2020;30(1):1–6.

23. Rassman William, Pak Jae. Follicular Unit Extraction: Evolution of a Technology. J Transplant Tech Res 2016;06. https://doi.org/10.4172/2161-0991. 1000158.

24. Garg AK, Garg S. Donor Harvesting: Follicular Unit Excision. J Cutan Aesthet Surg 2018;11(4):195–201.

25. Gabros S, Masood S. Central Centrifugal Cicatricial Alopecia. 2021. In: StatPearls [Internet]. Treasure Island (FL). StatPearls Publishing; 2022. PMID: 32644613.

26. Louis M, Travieso R, Oles N, et al. Narrative review of facial gender surgery: approaches and techniques for the frontal sinus and upper third of the face. Ann Transl Med 2021;9(7):606.

27. Epstein JS, Epstein GK, Epstein A, Brown R. Title: Hairline Lowering Surgery: Outcomes of 49 Consecutive Patients. Submitted for publication May 2022, Facial Plastic Surgery and Aesthetic Medicine.

Managing the Asian Eyelid

W. Katherine Kao, MD, Tang Ho, MD, MSc*

KEYWORDS

- Ethnic • Asian eyelid • Asian blepharoplasty • Double eyelid • Blepharoptosis • Brow ptosis

KEY POINTS

- The Asian eyelid differs anatomically from the Caucasian eyelid and special considerations should be taken into account when addressing the Asian eyelid.
- Patients seeking Asian blepharoplasty often seek enhancement of their ethnic features rather than occidentalization of the eyelid.
- Preoperative discussion should clarify the patient's esthetic goals and discuss the patient's desires for an upper eyelid crease.
- In the aging Asian eyelid, evaluation for blepharoptosis and discussion of concurrent blepharoptosis repair needs to be made.
- In the aging eyelid, infrabrow skin excision is a technique that can be considered in patients with excess lateral hooding and brow ptosis.

INTRODUCTION

The term "Asian" encompasses and refers to a diverse population with equally diverse ethnic features. Within this population, the eye is one of the most distinctive and defining features of the face imparting the patient with their ethnic identity. The Asian eyelid has some key defining features. These include the variable presence of a supratarsal fold or eyelid crease, a full upper eyelid appearance, epicanthal fold variability, and upward lateral canthal tilt. If a crease is present, there can be many variations in the configuration of the crease including variable crease height, contour, lateral flare, fold pattern, and variable relationship with the epicanthal fold. In the esthetic patient, even a small change in the upper eyelid crease can impart a dramatic change or improvement in facial appearance.

The Asian eyelid skin is often thicker than the eyelid skin in Caucasians. This can present a challenge to treatment and management when wide excision must be done to correct severe dermatochalasis. The brow position and relationship to the upper eyelid should also be determined. Blepharoptosis should also be carefully assessed for, as the redundant upper eyelid skin can mask underlying ptosis. Lastly, contrary to popular practice 20 to 30 years ago, patients of Asian descent largely desire an enhancement of their ethnic features rather than occidentalization of these features. The successful blepharoplasty surgeon will do well to understand this nuance when operating on the Asian upper eyelid.

ANATOMY

An understanding of key anatomic features of the Asian eyelid is essential to understanding the available approaches and techniques to surgical refinement and treatment of the Asian eyelid. The Asian upper eyelid often has a fuller appearance, variable configuration of the supratarsal fold, narrower palpebral fissure, variable degree of lash ptosis, upward lateral canthal tilt, and presence of an epicanthal fold.[1] The main anatomic feature accounting for the unique appearance of the Asian eyelid is the inferiorly displaced insertion of the orbital septum onto the levator aponeurosis[2,3] (**Fig. 1**). The insertion is lower in Asians than in Caucasians (**Fig. 2**). This lower insertion point causes the preaponeurotic fat pad to descend

Department of Otorhinolaryngology/Head and Neck Surgery, Texas Center for Facial Plastic Surgery, McGovern Medical School at the University of Texas Health Science Center in Houston, 6431 Fannin Street, MSB 5.036, Houston, TX 77030, USA
* Corresponding author.
E-mail address: tang.ho@uth.tmc.edu

Facial Plast Surg Clin N Am 30 (2022) 471–480
https://doi.org/10.1016/j.fsc.2022.07.009

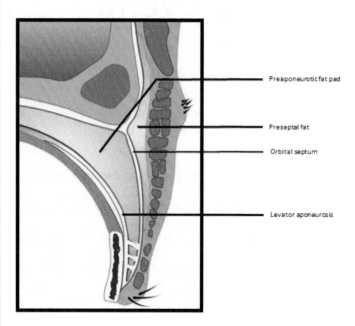

Preaponeurotic fat pad

Preseptal fat

Orbital septum

Levator aponeurosis

Fig. 1. *Asian eyelid anatomy*: This illustration of the Asian eyelid shows the low attachment of the orbital septum to the levator aponeurosis that blunts the attachments of the levator aponeurosis to the skin. This results in a variable eyelid crease and fuller eyelid appearance. Note the presence of a preseptal fat pad that is absent in the Caucasian eyelid.

along the levator aponeurosis which imparts a fullness to the Asian eyelid (see **Fig. 1**). This descent of preaponeurotic fat can also frequently blunt the aponeurotic attachments to the orbicularis muscle and upper eyelid skin. This accounts for either absence of the upper eyelid crease or lower eyelid crease height when compared with the Caucasian eyelid.[4]

Another key anatomic difference between the Asian and Caucasian eyelid is the continuity of the brow fat pad into the upper eyelid. In the Asian eyelid, the brow fat pad continues inferiorly in the preseptal/post-orbicularis muscle space and further contributes to the fullness in the appearance of the Asian upper eyelid (see **Fig. 1**). These fat pads may atrophy with age and contribute to a hollowed out and skeletonized look in the aging Asian eyelid.[2,3,5]

Eyelid Crease and the Epicanthal Fold

Depending on the study cited, approximately 50% of the Asian population has a visible supratarsal fold or eyelid crease.[6] The presence of this crease is referred to as a "double eyelid." The absence of a crease is referred to as a single eyelid or monolid (**Fig. 3**). The double eyelid is traditionally perceived to esthetically open the eye, impart a more feminine appearance to the eye and make the eye appear larger, although there is no change in the actual vertical palpebral fissure measurement. The double eyelid also allows the application of cosmetics to the tarsal platform. The creation of a double eyelid is referred to as "double eyelid

surgery" and has been one of the most popular procedures in Asia. However, placement of a high crease more anatomically consistent with a Caucasian eyelid can result in an unnatural and surprised look.[3,7]

The height of the Asian supratarsal fold varies between 6 to 8 mm in females and 4 to 6 mm in males.[8] This crease can be divided into three categories: (1) single eyelid (no eyelid crease), (2) low eyelid crease, and (3) double eyelid[1,9] (see **Fig. 3**). The double eyelid has been further described to run parallel to the ciliary margin, be partial or incomplete, and nasally tapered. Kiranantawat and colleagues[3] classified the double eyelid into three groups in relation to the epicanthal fold: (1) in-fold describes a lid crease that is lower than the epicanthal fold; (2) on-fold describes a lid crease that is right on the epicanthal fold; and (3) out-fold describes a crease that is higher than the epicanthal fold. The epicanthal fold is a semi-lunar fold of skin overlying the medial canthus region of the eye. It can have various anatomic configurations and has been classified into four different types: epicanthus supraciliaris, epicanthus palpebralis, epicanthus tarsalis, and epicanthus inversus. Epicanthus tarsalis, arising from the medial canthus and extending laterally, is the most common type seen in the Asian eyelid.[10,11]

PREOPERATIVE EVALUATION

The preoperative evaluation should include a discussion of the eyelid crease and whether or not it is desired. It is important to keep in mind that

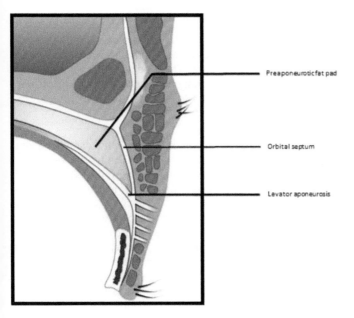

Fig. 2. *Caucasian eyelid anatomy*: In the Caucasian eyelid, the levator aponeurosis joins with the orbital septum and sends fibers to the skin of the eyelid to create the eyelid crease. There is no preaponeurotic fat layer in the Caucasian eyelid (see Asian eyelid illustration for comparison).

Preaponeuroticfat pad

Orbital septum

Levator aponeurosis

many Asian patients desire an enhancement of their ethnic characteristics and not a westernized look.[2,3,11] Discussion should include whether the patient would like the crease to be parallel to the ciliary margin or taper nasally to blend in with the epicanthal fold.[2,11,12] The contour of the eyelid crease and the degree of lateral flare should also be discussed. The proposed eyelid crease may be shown with a cotton-tipped applicator used to fold in the upper eyelid skin. Some patients who are adept at cosmeceutical application can show the desired lid appearance using commercially produced upper eyelid tape designed to create a temporary double eyelid fold. At the conclusion

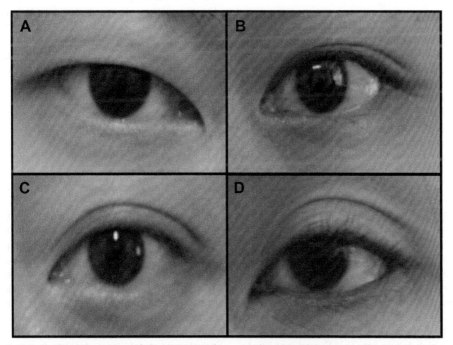

Fig. 3. *Variations in the appearance of the supratarsal crease*: There are variations in the supratarsal crease/eyelid crease. (*A*) Monolid, there is absence of an eyelid crease. (*B*) Eyelid crease blending medially with the epicanthal fold. (*C*) Eyelid crease running parallel to the epicanthal fold. (*D*) Multiple creases present.

of the visit, the patient and physician should both be clear regarding the desired appearance of the eyelid crease, height, contour, and features.

A full eye examination should also be conducted and include a full history and physical examination. History of dry eye, autoimmune disease, previous ophthalmic conditions, or surgery should be gathered. A comprehensive eye examination should be done to assess visual acuity, extraocular muscle motility, degree of dermatochalasis, presence of ptosis, brow position, presence of lash ptosis, fat pad prolapse, and lacrimal gland prolapse. Schirmer's test and the presence of Bell's phenomenon should also be assessed preoperatively; patients with dry eye will be at higher risk for exposure keratopathy following blepharoplasty procedures. Any existing asymmetry in the brow or eyelids should be pointed out to patients before any surgery. Preexisting ptosis should be evaluated for as well, as this can be addressed at the time of eyelid crease creation. Lifting the eyelid skin to analyze the true eyelid margin and levator function should be done.[2,11]

DOUBLE EYELID SURGERY

There are two broad technique categories for the creation of the upper eyelid crease. They are generally classified as closed (suture technique) or open (incision with or without skin excision).

Closed Technique

Suture techniques to create an upper eyelid crease were first described in 1896 by Mikamo.[13] It was subsequently refined in the latter half of the twentieth century and is still used by surgeons today. The technique uses intradermal sutures to anchor the orbicularis muscle and skin to the underlying levator aponeurosis or tarsal plate. To perform the technique, three sutures are placed along the length of the desired eyelid crease.[2,6,11–13] The desired upper eyelid crease is marked about 6 to 8 mm above the lid margin. The marking should agree with a preoperative discussion of the eyelid crease contour and height. Three points are marked along the eyelid crease medially, centrally, and laterally. Following injection of local anesthetic, the upper eyelid is everted, the superior tarsal border is identified and three double arm sutures are passed through the premarked points. The sutures are either externalized or buried underneath a stab incision. There are obvious limitations to the suture technique including a high failure rate[11,14,15] and inability to address dermatochalasis or shape the fat pads of the eye.

Open Technique

The open technique is the procedure of choice in upper eyelid crease formation and concurrent blepharoplasty. The open technique involves a skin incision that can simultaneously address dermatochalasis, ptosis, or fat pad prominence.

Skin marking

The open technique begins with a careful marking of the desired skin crease. The typical location of the esthetic Asian upper eyelid crease is about 6 to 8 mm above the lid margin but it can range from 3 to 10 mm.[2,6,11,12,16,17] An eyelid crease less than 6 mm high is typically reserved for patients who have a very narrow palpebral fissure and small orbital width. Medially, the eyelid crease should taper and blend to hide beneath the epicanthal fold. If the patient desires an epicanthoplasty, this medial mark should be adapted to the epicanthoplasty markings. If there is no epicanthal fold, the medial aspect of the marking can be positioned higher to create an upper eyelid crease that runs parallel to the lid margin. Laterally, the eyelid crease can have varying degrees of flare to suit the esthetic taste of the patient. Once the eyelid crease is marked, the amount of excess skin is determined using the pinch technique with a Green fixation forcep and marked for excision.

Surgical technique

Local anesthetic is injected and a blade is used to make the skin incisions. The skin and orbicularis oculi muscle are excised. The orbital septum is then identified and opened along the entire length of the incision from lateral to medial. The medial and central fat pads are identified and sculpted. Following contour and shaping of the fat pads, the distal aspect of the levator aponeurosis is identified along with the superior tarsal border. Suture fixation is performed to create the supratarsal crease. Three eyelid fixation sutures are then placed using a double-armed 6-0 prolene or nylon suture. The suture is passed through the skin, levator aponeurosis, and skin centrally (**Fig. 4**). The patient is then asked to open the eye to assess the position of the stitch. The medial and lateral sutures are then placed in a similar fashion and the incision is closed with subcuticular permanent suture. In the senior author's clinical experience, closure of the incision in the Asian eyelid is best done using a permanent suture in a subcuticular fashion. The Asian upper eyelid skin is thicker and more prone to hyperpigmentation and the development of train tracks from a running closure. For this reason, careful closure with 6-0 prolene subcuticular sutures is preferred.

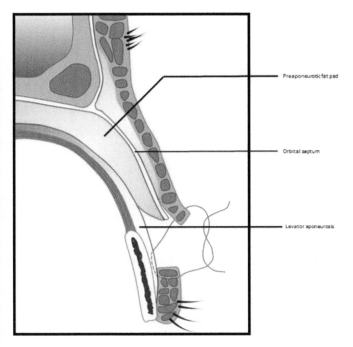

Preaponeurotic fat pad

Orbital septum

Levator aponeurosis

Fig. 4. *Suture fixation of the eyelid crease*: This illustration shows the suture fixation of the eyelid crease. The suture is passed through skin and orbicularis muscle, through the levator aponeurosis and again through skin and orbicularis before being tied down, allowing the levator to adhere to the skin and orbicularis oculi muscle, creating an upper eyelid crease.

MANAGEMENT OF THE AGING ASIAN EYELID

There are unique characteristics of the aging Asian eyelid that should be considered when selecting surgical approaches and techniques. The surgeon must keep in mind that the Asian eyelid skin is generally thicker than Caucasian eyelid skin. This may limit the degree of skin resection possible in a standard upper blepharoplasty approach to avoid an unnaturally thick and heavy appearance to the upper eyelid. In addition, blepharoptosis can often be masked by excessive hanging upper eyelid skin. Astute identification of blepharoptosis is important to avoid undesirable postoperative results.

Age-Related Changes in the Asian Eyelid

As the eyelid ages, dermatochalasis and volume loss result in hooding of the eyelid skin and camouflage of pretarsal show. In severe cases of dermatochalasis, the redundant upper eyelid skin may completely hide any pretarsal eyelid show and cause prolapse of the eyelashes which may lead to chronic blepharitis. The position of the brow laterally should also be noted, as severe brow ptosis laterally contributes to lateral hooding and lash ptosis. Orbital fat atrophy results in skeletonization of the orbital rim and an appearance of sunken upper eyelids.[18] The horizontal and vertical palpebral fissures decrease as well[19,20] and lastly, skeletal remodeling with resultant resorption of the

midface and superomedial orbital rim results in unwanted enophthalmos.[21]

Involutional blepharoptosis is often found in conjunction with the above-described changes. There are various causes of involutional ptosis with levator aponeurosis involvement seen in 90% of involutional ptosis cases.[21] The changes in the levator aponeurosis associated with involutional ptosis include levator dehiscence, disinsertion, attenuation, and fatty degeneration of the levator muscle. Characteristic changes in ptosis involve decreased margin reflex distance (MRD 1) measurement and increased pretarsal show. Enophthalmos resulting from skeletal remodeling of the bony orbit have also been associated with involutional ptosis. In upright position, an enophthalmic globe sits more caudally within the bony orbit resulting in progressive stretching of Whitnall's ligament resulting in eventual ptosis of the upper eyelid.[21]

Dermatochalasis versus blepharochalasis
Dermatochalasis and blepharochalasis are often confused with each other. Blepharochalasis is characterized by repeated episodic inflammation of the eyelids.[22,23] The symptoms were first described by Beer in 1807 but the term blepharochalasis was not attached to the condition until 1896 when Fuchs published a report of similar cases and attributed the term blepharochalasis to them.[22] The condition typically involves both upper eyelids but rare cases of lower eyelid

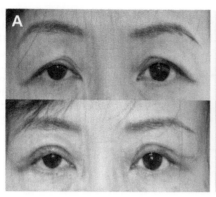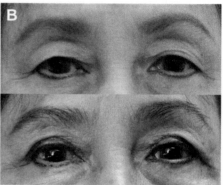

Fig. 5. *Upper blepharoplasty for dermatochalasis. (A and B)* Showing before and after results in two patients undergoing bilateral upper blepharoplasty for dermatochalasis. Note the improvement in lateral hooding and lash ptosis following blepharoplasty.

involvement or unilateral involvement have also been described. Blepharochalasis is characterized by an active and quiescent phase. In the active phase, patients experience recurrent episodes of nontender, nonpitting, nonerythematous edema of the upper eyelids generally refractory to antihistamines, and corticosteroids. The frequency of attacks is about three to four times per year but weekly episodes of edema have also been reported in the literature. As the patient ages, these episodes become less frequent and the condition enters a quiescent stage characterized by the lack of episodes for a minimum of 2 years. After several cycles of edema, the upper eyelid skin becomes paper thin, redundant, and baggy with tortuous vessels and visible telangiectasias.[22]

Dermatochalasis is an involutional change in the eyelid skin, whereas blepharochalasis is characterized by skin changes secondary to episodic stretching and deflation of the skin. Differentiating the two conditions is important because surgical repair techniques may vary in blepharochalasis. Timing of surgery will also have to be carefully considered in blepharochalasis with a quiescent period of 6 to 12 months recommended before surgery.[24,25]

Operative techniques for the aging upper eyelid

There are a few key factors that need to be considered when performing aging Asian blepharoplasty. The first is the placement of the incision lines. As described previously in this article, the esthetic upper eyelid crease in Asian patients, at 6 to 8 mm above the lid margin, is lower than it is in Caucasian patients. The amount of excised skin is often less than that of Westerners and fat removal should be conservative.[5]

In Asian eyelids, the difference in thickness between the supratarsal and infrabrow regions is more significant than in Caucasians. This anatomic difference is responsible for the unnatural results from Westernization blepharoplasties in the past. Because pretarsal skin is thinner than infrabrow skin, wide skin excision required in excessive lateral hooding results in the closure of thin pretarsal skin to the thicker upper eyelid/infrabrow skin. The thicker infrabrow skin then falls over the newly created eyelid crease resulting in a thickened upper eyelid fold that looks unnatural.[2,5,26] Care should also be taken to minimize the lateral extension and lateral excision of excess skin.[27] Extension of the upper blepharoplasty scar beyond the lateral canthus can result in a prominent and unnaturally appearing scar.[26] Asian skin is more prone to hyperpigmentation and this lateral extension is often poorly camouflaged due to the healing characteristics of Asian skin types.

Upper blepharoplasty technique The upper blepharoplasty technique begins with a proper marking of the upper eyelid crease. The crease should sit between 6 and 8 mm above the lid margin and taper medially to blend in with the epicanthal fold, if one is present. The medial aspect of the incision should not extend beyond the medial canthus to prevent scar contracture and unnatural results. Laterally, the incision line should not extend more than 1 cm laterally from the lateral canthus to avoid a prominent looking scar. Once the upper eyelid crease is marked, the amount of redundant skin is determined using the skin pinch technique. Conservative excision is favored in Asian patient.

Once the incision lines are marked, local anesthetic is infiltrated and a blade is used to excise skin and orbicularis oculi muscle. The orbital septum is then incised to expose the orbital fat pads. These are sculpted and debulked where needed. In patients with an existing upper eyelid

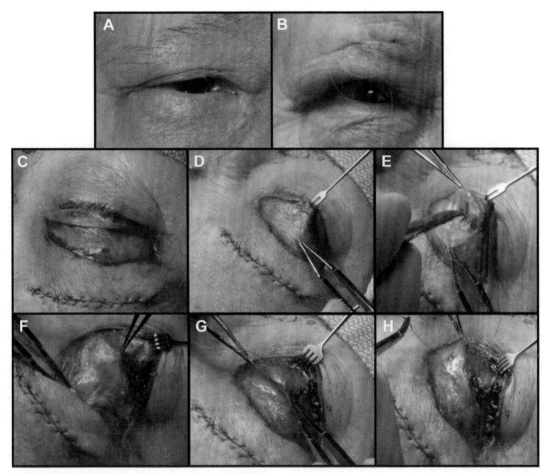

Fig. 6. *External blepharoptosis repair:* This series of intraoperative pictures shows the dissection involved when performing the external approach to blepharoptosis repair. (*A*) Preoperative photo showing low MRD1 and right upper eyelid ptosis. (*B*) Postoperative photo showing correction of blepharoptosis. (*C*) Blepharoplasty completed, the skin and orbicularis have been removed and the orbital septum is visible. (*D*) The orbital septum is entered and the preaponeuroic fat pad (yellow) is encountered. (*E*) The preaponeurotic fat is lifted and dissection posterior to the preaponeurotic fat is carried out to expose the levator aponeurosis. (*F*) The preaponeurotic fat is retracted and the levator aponeurosis is now fully visible. The levator aponeurosis is then dissected posteriorly to free it up adequately for advancement and fixation. (*G*) A prolene suture is passed through the tarsal plate. (*H*) The suture is then passed through the levator aponeurosis and secured, thus correcting the blepharoptosis.

crease, closure can then be done at this point. In patients who desire an upper eyelid crease, the "double eyelid" can be created at this point by dissecting and identifying the levator aponeurosis. The levator aponeurosis is then sutured to the tarsal plate and upper eyelid skin using three double-armed permanent sutures. One eyelid crease suture is placed centrally, one is placed medially and the last is placed laterally. Following the creation of the upper eyelid crease, the eyelid incision is closed using a 6-0 prolene subcuticular suture to prevent train tracking and minimize postoperative scarring (**Fig. 5**).

Ptosis management/technique There are two main approaches to address ptosis in the upper eyelid, an anterior or posterior approach. Because the aging eyelid patient will often require skin excision at the time of surgery, the anterior approach is often done. Following resection of skin and orbicularis oculi muscle, the superior border of the tarsal plate is identified along with the orbital septum. The orbital septum is then entered and the preaponeurotic fat is identified. The preaponeurotic fat is then lifted to reveal the levator aponeurosis. The levator aponeurosis is then sutured to the tarsal border using a double arm 5-0 or 6-0 prolene suture (**Fig. 6**). Various points of fixation are required depending on individual patient characteristics. The patient is then asked to open the eye and the eyelid height is assessed. Adjustment in levator fixation to the tarsal plate can be made at

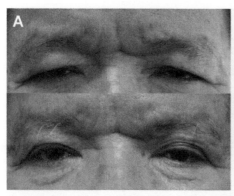
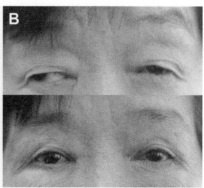

Fig. 7. *Bilateral infrabrow skin excision blepharoplasty (IBEB) for dermatochalasis*: (*A and B*) Showing before and after results of two patients undergoing IBEB for heavy dermatochalasis and lateral hooding. Note the well camouflaged incision postoperatively and significant improvement in dermatochalasis and lateral hooding without significant unsightly scarring or disturbance to the upper eyelid crease.

this point to restore the height and establish symmetry.[19,21]

Infrabrow skin excision blepharoplasty The infrabrow skin excision blepharoplasty (IBEB) has become more widely used in the management of the Asian aging eyelid. As mentioned previously, in patients who have severe dermatochalasis and lateral hooding, the adequate correction will necessitate the removal of a wide area of excess skin with lateral extension to address the lateral hooding component. This wide excision results in reapproximation of the thicker infrabrow skin with the thinner pretarsal skin. This can lead to an unnatural appearance in the upper eyelid with bunching and prolapse of the heavier infrabrow skin over the newly created crease. Second, lateral extension results in a conspicuous scar that extends beyond the lateral canthus. In patients who do not desire a separate browpexy or brow lift procedure, an infrabrow skin excision may be preferable.[26,28,29]

IBEB is straightforward to perform and avoids manipulation of the existing eyelid crease. Surgical excision begins with marking a line along the ciliary margin of the eyebrow. This will form the superior aspect of the skin excision. The incision should start about 2 to 3 mm laterally from the medial aspect of the brow. Following marking of the inferior edge of the eyebrow, forceps are used to pinch the skin and determine the amount of excess skin to be resected. The greatest width of skin excised from the lateral eyelid should not exceed 8 to 12 mm.[29] Following marking, a blade is used to make an incision along the previously marked lines. The blade is positioned at a 30° angle, parallel to the direction of the hair follicles to prevent transection and injury to the hair follicles. Cautery can then be used to dissect and

excise skin, subcutaneous fat, and orbicularis oculi muscle. The results of the IBEB can deliver good correction of severe dermatochalasis (**Fig. 7**) without disruption of the eyelid crease and without accentuation of "crow's feet" along the lateral orbital rim.

Brow management There are several techniques that can be used to address brow ptosis. These include the direct brow lift, browpexy, coronal brow lift, pretrichial brow lift, temporal brow lift, and endoscopic brow lift. A comprehensive review of brow lift techniques is beyond the scope of this article, however, the browpexy technique will be reviewed as this is easily performed concurrently at the time of blepharoplasty and can be done without making another incision.

Browpexy can be done at the same time as upper eyelid blepharoplasty. Following adequate excision of skin and orbicularis muscle, the orbicularis oculi muscle is retracted and blunt dissection is used to expose the brow retaining ligaments. Once the brow retaining ligaments are identified, they are cut, resulting in release of the lateral and central brow. The deep galea and orbital ligament are then incised to expose the brow fat pad laterally. Blunt dissection is continued beyond the orbital rim along the periosteum. The brow fat pad is then sculpted and suspended to the periosteum approximately 1 to 2 cm above the lateral orbital rim with permanent suture. This technique ensures the brow fat pad and not the frontalis muscle is fixated to the periosteum to avoid restriction and limitation in the frontalis muscle during elevation and facial animation of the brow.[30]

SUMMARY

The Asian eyelid is a complex subunit with distinct appearance and characteristics. Surgical enhancement of the Asian eyelid should be carried out with delicate precision. Key aspects in the analysis and treatment of the Asian eyelid include preoperative discussion of the eyelid crease. The eyelid crease in Asian patients should sit lower than in Caucasian patients. Careful design of the eyelid crease with this in mind will minimize the risk of an unnatural appearance. The aging Asian eyelid also has unique characteristics to consider. Because the skin of the Asian eyelid is thicker and because there is a significant difference in thickness of the infrabrow skin and pretarsal skin, consideration should be made to minimize the width and lateral extent of skin excision to maintain a natural result. In patients with significant brow ptosis and lateral hooding, a browpexy, direct brow lift or IBEB skin excision can be considered. With these points and elements in mind, functional and esthetic improvement can be achieved in the Asian blepharoplasty patient.

CLINICS CARE POINTS

- The Asian eyelid is anatomically different from the Caucasian eyelid
- The goal of Asian upper blepharoplasty is enhancement of ethnic features rather than occidentalization of the upper eyelid
- Preoperative discussion should clarify the patient's desires regarding a supratarsal crease and the contour of the double eyelid
- Blepharoptosis should be evaluated at the time of consultation
- Infrabrow skin excision can be a valuable tool in the aging eyelid, especially in cases with brow ptosis and significant lateral hooding.

DISCLOSURE

W.K. Kao has no financial disclosures to report. T. Ho is medical director for Hansbiomed USA, Inc.

REFERENCES

1. Saonanon P. Update on Asian eyelid anatomy and clinical relevance. Curr Opin Ophthalmol 2014; 25(5):436–42. Available at: https://pubmed.ncbi. nlm.nih.gov/24852200/.
2. Lee KJ, Karam AM, Lam SM. Modern Advances in Asian Blepharoplasty. In: Massry Guy, Murphy Mark R, Azizzadeh B, editors. Master techniques in blepharoplasty and Periorbital Rejuvenation. New York: Springer New York LLC; 2011. p. 147–56.
3. Kiranantawat K, Suhk JH, Nguyen AH. The Asian Eyelid: Relevant Anatomy. Semin Plast Surg 2015; 29(3):158–64.
4. Kakizaki H, Leibovitch I, Selva D, et al. Orbital septum attachment on the levator aponeurosis in Asians: in vivo and cadaver study. Ophthalmology 2009;116(10):2031–5.
5. Park DD. Aging Asian Upper Blepharoplasty and Brow. Semin Plast Surg 2015;29(3):188–200.
6. Nguyen MQ, Hsu PW, Dinh TA. Asian Blepharoplasty. Semin Plast Surg 2009;23(3):185–97.
7. Chen WP. What is an Upper Lid Crease?. In: Asian blepharoplasty and the eyelid crease. Amsterdam, Netherlands: Elsevier Inc; 2016. p. 1–15.
8. Liu D, Hsu W. Oriental eyelids. Anatomic difference and surgical consideration. Ophthalmic Plast Reconstr Surg 1986;2(2):59–64.
9. Jeong S, Lemke B, Dortzbach R, et al. The Asian upper eyelid: an anatomical study with comparison to the Caucasian eyelid. Arch Ophthalmol 1999; 117(7):907–12.
10. Chen W.P., Comparative Anatomy of the Eyelids, In: Asian blepharoplasty and the eyelid Crease2, Elsevier Inc; Amsterdam, Netherlands, 19–38.
11. Weng C-J. Oriental Upper Blepharoplasty. Semin Plast Surg 2009;23(1):5–15.
12. Lee CK, Ahn ST, Kim N. Asian Upper Lid Blepharoplasty. Clin Plast Surg 2013;40:167–78.
13. Alameddine Ramzi m, Lee BW, Lu W, et al. Aesthetic Rejuvenation in the Patient of Asian Ancestry. In: Azizzadeh B, Murphy MR, Johnson CM, et al, editors. Master techniques in facial Rejuvenation. Amsterdam, Netherlands: Elsevier Inc; 2018. p. 166–72.
14. Mutou Y, Mutou H. Intradermal double eyelid operation and its follow-up results. Br J Plast Surg 1972; 25(3):285–91.
15. Homma K, Mutou Y, Muout H, et al. Intradermal stitch blepharoplasty for orientals: does It disappear? Aesthetic Plast Surg 2000;24(4):289–91.
16. Kruavit A. Asian Blepharoplasty: An 18-year Experience in 6215 Patients. Aesthet Surg J 2009;29(4): 272–83.
17. Chen WPD. Asian Upper Blepharoplasty. JAMA Facial Plast Surg 2018;20(3):249–50.
18. Liang L, Sheha H, Fu Y, et al. Ocular surface morbidity in eyes with senile sunken upper eyelids. Ophthalmology 2011;118(12):2487–92.
19. Guyuron B, Harvey D. Periorbital and Orbital Aging: Senile Enophthalmos as a Cause of Upper Eyelid Ptosis. Plast Reconstr Surg 2016;138(1): 31e–7e.
20. Park DH, Choi WS, Yoon SH, et al. Anthropometry of asian eyelids by age. Plast Reconstr Surg 2008; 121(4):1405–13.

21. Lee T-Y, Shin YH, Lee JG. Strategies of upper blepharoplasty in aging patients with involutional ptosis. Arch Plast Surg. 2020;47(4):290–6.

22. Koursh DM, Modjtahedi SP, Selva D, et al. The Blepharochalasis Syndrome. Surv Ophthalmol 2009; 54(2):235–44.

23. Zhou J, Ding J, Li D. Blepharochalasis: clinical and epidemiological characteristics, surgical strategy and prognosis – a retrospective cohor study with 93 cases. BMC Ophthalmol 2021;21:313–9.

24. Bergin D, McCord C, Berger T, et al. Blepharochalasis. Br J Ophthalmol 1988;72(11):863–7.

25. Collin J. Blepharochalasis. A review of 30 cases. Ophthalmic Plast Reconstr Surg 1991;7(3):153–7.

26. Osaki MH, Osaki TH, Osaki T. Infrabrow Skin Excision Associated with Upper Blepharoplasty to Address Significant Dermatochalasis with Lateral Hooding in Select Asian Patients. Ophthalmic Plast Reconstr Surg 2017;1:53–6.

27. Cho I. Aging Blepharoplasty. Arch Plast Surg 2013; 40(5):486–91.

28. Lee YJ, Kim S, Lee J, et al. Parallel-excision infrabrow blepharoplasty with extensive excision of the orbicularis oculi muscle in an Asian population. 2archives Plast Surg 2020;47(2):171–7.

29. Sugamata A. Infraeyebrow Blepharoplasty for Blepharochalasis of the Upper Eyelid: It's Indication and Priority. Plast Surg Int 2012;1–5.

30. Georgescu D, Belsare G, McCann JD, et al. Adjunctive Procedures in Upper Eyelid Blepharoplasty: Internal Brow Fat Sculpting and Elevation, Glabellar Myectomy , and Lacrimal Gland Repositioning. In: Massry G, Murphy MR, Azizzadeh B, editors. *Master Techniques in Blepharoplasty and Periorbital Rejuvenation*. New York: Springer; 2011. p. 101–8.

Buccal Fat Reduction
Indications, Surgical Techniques, Complications

Jorge A. Espinosa Reyes, MD[a],*, Juan Gabriel Camacho Triana, MD[b]

KEYWORDS

- Buccal fat pad removal • Bichectomy • Surgical technique • Intraoral approach

KEY POINTS

- This article describes the technique of intraoral removal of the buccal fat pad.
- Anatomy knowledge and careful surgical technique are the primary considerations for a successful procedure with a low incidence of complications.
- The technique's main characteristics are the intraoral approach using blunt dissection and suction-assisted buccal fat pad extraction.

 Video content accompanies this article at http://www.facialplastic.theclinics.com.

INTRODUCTION

The image of the face is the primary source of information for the viewer regarding age, health, and race in nonverbal communication (Video 1). As one of the goals for most people is to look younger and more attractive, the tools and procedures that facial plastic surgeons have to modify these shapes and features are one of the most appreciated resources.

The buccal fat pad, or Bichat fat pad, is an adipose structure on the cheeks, first identified by the German Laurentius Heister, who considered it a gland. In 1802, the Frenchman Marie François Xavier Bichat found that its nature was adipose tissue. This structure relates to the chewing muscles and acts as a cushion between them.[1] Bichat's fat pad is located between the anterior margin of the masseter and the buccinator, with the mean volumetric variation found to be 7.8 to 11.2 mL for males and 7.2 to 10.8 mL for females, with a mean thickness of 6 mm. Imaging studies demonstrate that the buccal fat pad grows significantly from ages 10 to 20, increasing from 4000 to 8000 cubic millimeters, then declining in size over the next 30 years to an average volume of 7000 cubic millimeters.[2]

In some people, the presence of a sizable fatty volume may result in a rounded face, creating a disharmonious facial contour and the impression of being overweight.[1]

The change in volume, increasing or lowering the size of the malar bones, the chin, the lips, and the mandibula, as well as the reduction in the volume of the descended jowls, the cheeks, and the neck, can make a person look younger, thinner, more balanced, and more attractive. In addition, other procedures, such as refining the nose, eyes, lips, and neck are keys in the search for a more balanced and harmonic face.

Removing the buccal fat pad is one of the most straightforward procedures to attain this goal.[1,2] Nevertheless, the right choice of the patient regarding age, body weight, and expectations can make a profound difference in the result of the surgery and the patient's satisfaction. Before surgery, the surgeon should consider the risks and possible complications. This procedure can be done as a unique surgery, but most of the

a Facial Plastic Surgeon, Calle 127a # 7- 53 cons 3005, Bogota, Colombia 110111; b Calle 121 # 53a -02, Bogota, Colombia 110111
* Corresponding author.
E-mail address: jorgespinosa@gmail.com

Facial Plast Surg Clin N Am 30 (2022) 481–488
https://doi.org/10.1016/j.fsc.2022.07.003

time, it is part of a more complex procedure involving the change of the other shapes of the face, such as the nose, chin, eyebrows, eyelids, and jowls, among others.

Multiple anatomic structures organized in layers and compartments determine the shape of the face going from the skin to the bone frame.[3] Immediately deep into the skin, the superficial fat pads homogenize the face's surface and cover the muscles, while the deeper compartments show the viewer the mimic of the emotions, age, health, and race. Under this superficial fat layer lays a muscle aponeurotic layer composed of the galea in the frontal area, the superficial temporal aponeurosis in the temporal area, the superficial musculoaponeurotic system (SMAS) in the cheek, and the platysma in the neck (**Fig. 1**).

Under this musculoaponeurotic layer, we find the deeper facial muscles, the mastication muscles, and the deep fat compartments.

The buccal extension of the buccal fat pad is part of a series of deep fat components that can affect the shape of the face, making it look fuller and rounded as if the patient were overweight, even if the patient has an average body mass index. The resection of this buccal extension can profoundly impact the shape and appearance of the face, making the patient look thinner and more athletic. Therefore, this procedure is one of the most frequently asked procedures in plastic surgery consultation.

The buccal fat pad is an adipose pillow located in the cheek and has a body with three lobes, each with its own capsule and blood supply. The posterior lobule has four extensions: the buccal, the pterygoid, the pterygopalatine, and the temporal[1,2,4–11]. The buccal extension and body account for roughly 50% of the buccal fat pad volume.[2]

The surgical modification of the buccal extension, which receives vascularization from the middle facial artery, can most affect the appearance of the face. This buccal extension is located superficial to the buccinator muscle and deep to the parotid masseteric fascia, the facial nerve, sand parotid duct[2,4] (**Fig. 2**).

The pterygopalatine extension goes to the pterygopalatine fossa. The pterygoid extension goes to the pterygoid-mandibular space, medial to the mandibular ramus, and surrounds the pterygoid muscles, and the temporal extension has a deep and superficial portion. The superficial portion lies between the temporalis muscle and its deep temporal fascia. It travels around the muscle to occupy the medial space next to the temporal muscle, receiving the name of the deep portion[2,4] The buccal fat pad has a volume described earlier,

and this does not change with changes in the patient's body weight.[4]

FUNCTION

For centuries, anatomists have studied the complex nature of pockets of fat on the face and attributed many functions to the buccal fat pad. One of the functions of the buccal fat pad is to facilitate gliding between the muscles of mastication. It also increases the resistance of the cheek during oral negative pressure nursing of the child (this explains the large volume of the buccal fat pad in infants and less volume in adults) and also protects the neurovascular bundles and the parotid duct. The other function is to give volume to the cheeks, affecting the esthetics of the face.[2,4,12]

INDICATIONS

The diagnosis is purely clinical, and it is not necessary to use X- Rays or tomography images to plan the procedure. The buccal fat pad removal is one of the procedures indicated when the aim is to make a face look thinner. It can be combined with the double chin reduction through neck lift surgery or submental liposuction, with the face liposuction, or the increase of the malar bones' size to achieve a more stylized looking face and a more triangular face shape. This triangular face shape is often related to youth and attractiveness in the face.[7]

The patient's age is a significant factor when discussing surgery indications. Most younger patients below the age of 20 years have a rounded face, which is characteristic of the childhood face. This shape will change with aging, resembling a more adult face with the lowering of the volume of the cheeks and the hardening of the facial features that come with adulthood. If the surgeon decides to extract the buccal fat pad in this age group, they should be aware that when the patient gets older, they can have a tired look and a significantly hollowed face.[7] Only patients with a very rounded face, full of volume in the cheeks, will improve their image, getting a younger and more elegantly defined face and maintaining this look with the passage of time.

Older patients, over the 30s, have an entirely developed face and have a more predictable result after the buccal fat pad removal. The only changes they will have in the future will be related to the aging process and the changes in their body weight. Of these patients, the ones with a full rounded face are fantastic candidates for the buccal fat pad removal, as they will achieve a more thin and elegant appearance after the surgery.

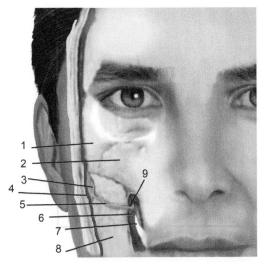

Fig. 1. Anatomy of the buccal fat pad, coronal schematic view. 1. Malar bone, 2. Maxillary bone, 3. Parotid gland, 4. SMAS, 5. Parotid duct, 6. Vestibular mucosa and buccinator muscle, 7. Vestibular space, and 8. Buccal fat pad, the relationship with the malar bone, and the SMAS.

However, the surgeon can get the best results in patients with an average corporal mass index who present a fully round face with excess volume in the middle cheek area.

In older patients with jowl descent as a result of the aging process, to prevent false expectations, the surgeon should be aware that jowls will not be affected with the removal of the buccal fat pad and explain it to the patient. In addition, there are different ways to correct them, such as facelift surgery or facial liposuction.

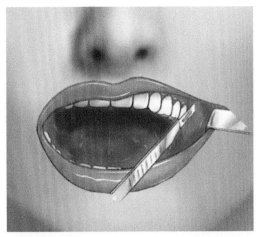

Fig. 3. The incision in the gingivobuccal sulcus 1 cm posterior and inferior to the parotid duct mucosal opening.

In the patient's diagnosis, it is of paramount importance that there be photo documentation. Besides the usual lateral, frontal, basal, and cenital (helicopter) views, the pictures taken with an upper light source can show the shape of the cheeks and the shadows of the malar bones better. Furthermore, to be able to show the patient the result of the surgery, the postoperative pictures should receive the exact source of light in the same set.

To approach the patient's outcome after the surgery, the doctor can use a mirror and ask the patient to suck the cheeks with their mouth closed. This maneuver will produce a cheek depression

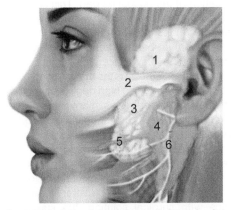

Fig. 2. Anatomy of the buccal fat pad, lateral schematic view showing the temporal extension and its relationship with the parotid duct and buccinator muscle. 1. Buccal fat pad temporal extension, 2. Zygomatic arch, 3. Buccal fat pad, 4. Parotid gland, 5. Parotideal gland, and 6. Facial nerve.

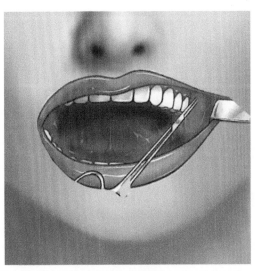

Fig. 4. With a closed, thinned point of a Kelly Adson clamp, the surgeon should apply a gentle pressure perpendicular to the mucosal plane.

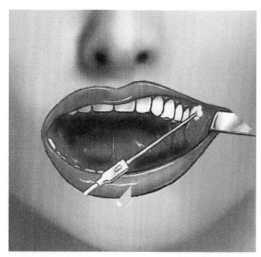

Fig. 5. The use of the suction of the cannula will pull out the fat quickly and with minimal manipulation of the surrounding structures.

in the place of the buccal fat pad and can be used to explain to the patient what results they can expect after the surgery and the extraction of the fat.

Therefore, buccal fat pad removal is a helpful technique to sculpt the angles of the face and enhance esthetics in patients with rounded faces, highlighting the malar and mandibular prominence.

Malar hypoplasia is not an indication for buccal fat pad removal. Buccal fat pad removal in these patients will result in a hollow appearance in their cheeks. For this reason, it is essential to

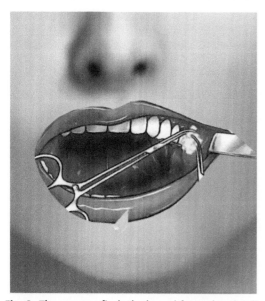

Fig. 6. The surgeon finds the buccal fat pad and pulls it by the suction cannula, can use two clamps to help with the extraction.

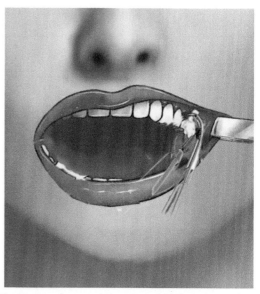

Fig. 7. On rare occasions, it is necessary to use cautery if the surgeon identifies a vessel in the buccal fat pedicle.

understand that buccal fat pad removal is not a substitute for malar augmentation.[2]

The surgeon should avoid doing this procedure on pregnant or lactating patients, patients with chronic illnesses, patients on blood-thinning agents, and patients younger than 18 years. In addition, it is important to understand that some fullness of the anteromedial portion of the face area result from the malar prominence and the posterolateral fullness may be due to masseter hypertrophy.[13]

The intraoral is the most systematic approach for buccal fat pad removal.[7] Therefore, it is critical for the procedure to know the anatomy and the exact location of the buccal fat pad. This knowledge will lead to a fast procedure with the lowest possible complications. Most of the time, it is better to do the buccal fat pad extraction under light sedation because the only place the surgeon can block with local anesthesia is the oral mucosa, and pulling the fat can produce a high degree of discomfort for the patient. Nevertheless, many patients desire this procedure done simultaneously with other facial procedures, such as rhinoplasty, mentoplasty, face liposuction, facelift, or submental volume reduction. Generally, in these cases, general anesthesia or local sedation is the usual choice.[7,12]

In the intraoral approach, after cleaning the surface with surgical solution, the surgeon should mark the incision in the gingivobuccal sulcus 1 cm posterior and inferior to the parotid duct mucosal opening. Usually, only a 5 mm incision made with the tip of an 11 blade is enough to take out the fat pad (**Fig. 3**). Then, with the closed,

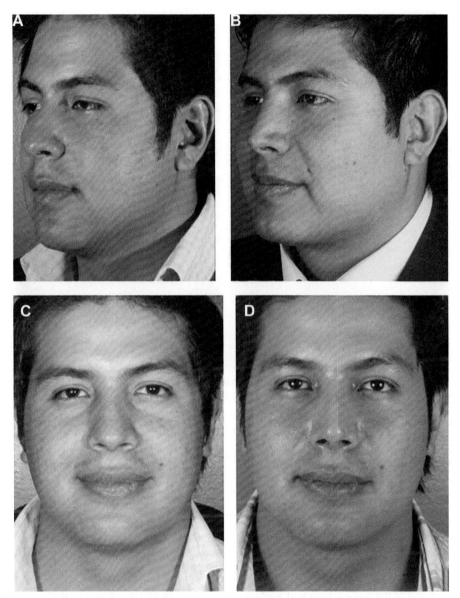

Fig. 8. Male patient buccal fat pad removal. (*A*) Pre-op oblique view. (*B*) Pop 3 months oblique view. (*C*) Pre-op frontal view. (*D*) Pop 3 months frontal view.

thin point of a Kelly Adson clamp, the surgeon should apply a gentle pressure perpendicular to the mucosal plane. The surgeon will feel when the clamp tip goes through the buccinator muscle, anterior to the anterior border of the masseter muscle, arriving at the pocket that contains the buccal fat pad (**Fig. 4**). The surgeon will feel the "click" or the change in the pressure when it goes through the buccinator muscle and, with the nondominant hand, can guide direction by feeling the masseter muscle's position. After this, without removing the Kelly Adson clamp, a gentle opening of its tip will let the surgeon insert a 10 Frasier suction cannula between the two valves,

reaching the fat pad pocket (**Fig. 5**). The buccal fat pad is the less resistant structure. The suction of the cannula will pull out the fat quickly and with minimal manipulation of the surrounding structures. This maneuver will diminish the risk of damaging the facial nerve, parotid duct, and facial vessels, which will be at risk. Once the surgeon finds the buccal fat pad and pulls it by the suction cannula, he or she can use two clamps to help with the extraction (**Fig. 6**). On rare occasions, it is necessary to use cautery if the surgeon identifies a vessel in the buccal fat pedicle (**Fig. 7**). The surgeon can extract all the fat from the right-selected patient. The usual fat volume extracted is between

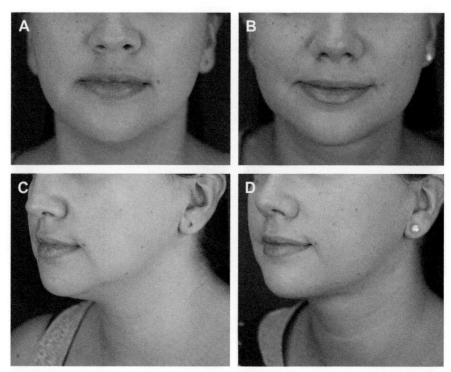

Fig. 9. Female patient buccal fat pad removal. (*A*) Pre-op oblique view. (*B*) Pop 3 months oblique view. (*C*) Pre-op frontal view. (*D*) Pop 3 months frontal view.

3 and 5 cc on each side and is stored in two 5 or 10 cc syringes to show to the patient after the surgery.[13] It is not usually necessary to use drains, and one 6 to 0 Vicryl stitch is usually enough to close the incision.

The facelift approach is the other approach to removing the buccal fat pad[7,12] The fat pad can be extracted laterally instead of the medial extraction of the intraoral approach. The surgical instruments will pass through this approach between the facial nerve buccal branches, blood vessels, and the parotid duct anterior to the masseter muscle. The exact use of the Kelly Adson and suction clamp technique can reduce the manipulation risk of this complex area.

COMPLICATIONS

Buccal fat pad reduction is generally considered a safe and relatively simple procedure. Complications related to buccal fat pad extraction are rare but clinically significant when they do occur. The buccal fat pad is close to multiple vessels, the facial nerve, and the parotid duct. Removal of the buccal fat pad can damage these vital structures. Complication rates are between 8.45% and 18%.[2]

The potential complications of the buccal fat pad resection are excessive bleeding, hematoma, facial buccal and zygomatic branch nerve lesions, parotid duct impairment, trismus, facial asymmetry, and infection.[2,4–8,12,14,15]

Adequate knowledge of anatomy and careful looking for the fat pack pocket with the minimal manipulation possible is critical to prevent it. In addition, appropriate informed consent is critical, considering that even if the surgeon performs an excellent surgical technique, complications can occur because of the intimate association of the buccal fat pad with vital structures.

POSTOPERATIVE INDICATIONS

After the surgery, there is no need for solid analgesics, and only acetaminophen is necessary. The prescription of chlorhexidine mouthwash and mild repose during the first 3 days is enough. Usually, there is no need for bandages. The results are usually evident after 2 weeks of the procedure, and the patient usually refers to high satisfaction.

SUMMARY

The refinement of the face looking for a chiseled and athletic image is one of the most frequent consultations in facial plastic surgery. Many procedures can help achieve this look, such as increasing malar and mandibular size with fillers or implants, face and neck liposuction, platysmal

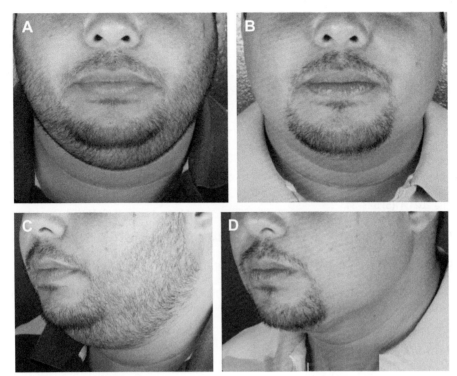

Fig. 10. Male patient buccal fat pad removal. (*A*) Pre-op oblique view. (*B*) Pop 3 months oblique view. (*C*) Pre-op frontal view. (*D*) Pop 3 months frontal view.

plication surgery, and resection of the subplatysmal fat and the buccal fat pad. The buccal fat pad resection is one of the best tools the surgeon has to achieve this result (**Figs. 8–10**).

Good patient selection and careful surgical technique are keys to a successful result. The fast recovery time, the perception of being a minor surgery, and the good results make the buccal fat pad resection one of the first options for doctors and patients.

The surgeon must remember that this fat is closely related to critical structures, such as the parotid duct, the facial nerve branches, and the facial vessels, so anatomic knowledge becomes a must in the surgery.

CLINICS CARE POINTS

- The anatomy is a key knowledge for the adecuate and safe treatment of thge buccal fat pad.
- The buccal fat pad removal is a key procedure in order to make the face look thiner and is a very good complement for other facial procedures in selected patients.

DISCLOSURE

The authors have nothing to disclose.

SUPPLEMENTARY DATA

Supplementary data related to this article can be found online at https://doi.org/10.1016/j.fsc.2022.07.003.

REFERENCES

1. Assunção Calixto Da Silva Diego, De Lucas Da Silva Almeida Fabio, Melo Nunes Ota Tamara, et al. Effects of Dexamethasone and Photobiomodulation on Pain, Swelling, and Quality of Life After Buccal Fat Pad Removal: A Clinical Trial. J Oral Maxillofac Surg Pág 2020;78(11).
2. Echlin Kezia, Whitehouse Harry, Schwaiger Michael, et al. A Cadaveric Study of the Buccal Fat Pad: Implications for Closure of Palatal Fistulae and Donor-Site Morbidity. Plast Reconstr Surg 2020;146(6): 1331–9.
3. Ozan Bitik. Commentary on: External Approach to Buccal Fat Excision in Facelift: Anatomy and Technique. Aesthet Surg J 2021;41.
4. Chouikh Fairouz, Dierks Eric J. The Buccal Fat Pad Flap. Oral Maxillofac Surg Clin North Am 2021;33(2).

5. Cral WG. The Importance of Ultrasound in Excision of the Buccal Fat Pad. Aesthetic Plast Surg 2021; 46(2):1007–8.

6. Pimentel Thais, Hadad Henrique, Statkievicz Cristian, et al. Management of Complications Related to Removal of the Buccal Fat Pad. J Craniofac Surg; 2021.

7. Moura L-B, Spin J-R, Spin-Neto R, et al. Buccal fat pad removal to improve facial aesthetics: an established technique? Med Oral Patol Oral Cir Bucal 2018;23(4):e478–84.

8. Surek CC, et al. External Approach to Buccal Fat Excision in Facelift: Anatomy and Technique. Aesthet Surg J 2021;41(5):527–34.

9. de Sena YRB, Rabêlo PMS, Gonçalves LM, et al. Comparison of Bichectomy Techniques Through a Clinical Case and 6-Month Follow-up. J Lasers Med Sci 2022;15(13):e2. https://doi.org/10.34172/jlms.2022.02.

10. Davis B, Serra M. Buccal fat pad reduction. s.l. : StatPearls [Internet]. Treasure Island (FL): StatPearls Publishing; 2022.

11. Grillo R, de la Puente Dongo JL, de Moura Moreira L, et al. Effectiveness of bandage in the incidence of major complications on bichectomy: literature review and case series of 643 bichectomies. Oral Maxillofac Surg 2021. https://doi.org/10.1007/s10006-021-01008-z.

12. Traboulsi-Garet B, Camps-Font O, Traboulsi-Garet M, et al. Buccal fat pad excision for cheek refinement: A systematic review. Med Oral Patol Oral Cir Bucal 2021.

13. Lip Ng C, Rival R, Solomon P. A Simple Technique to Measure the Volume of Removed Buccal Fat. Aesthet Surg J 2020;40(8):NP461–3.

14. Lin MJ, Hazan E, John AM, et al. Buccal Fat Pad Reduction With Intraoperative Fat Transfer to the Temple. Cutis. 2022;109(1):46–8.

15. Pokrowiecki R. Extended buccal lipectomy (bichectomy) for extreme cheek contouring. Int J Oral Maxillofac Surg 2022;51(7):929–32.

Face and Neck Lift Options in Patients of Ethnic Descent

David Edward James Whitehead, MBBS, BSc, MSc, FRCS(ORL-HNS)[a],*,
Özcan Çakmak, MD[b]

KEYWORDS

- MeSH • Rhytidoplasty • Cervicoplasty • Ethnicity • Aging
- Superficial musculo-aponeurotic system

KEY POINTS

- There is a significant ongoing shift in the utilization of cosmetic procedures across ethnicities.
- The most noticeable changes with age occur in all ethnicities over the mobile superficial musculo-aponeurotic system.
- Extended facelift techniques are most effective across all ethnicities by releasing the retaining ligaments.
- The complete release of the retaining ligaments of the midface and neck will facilitate the effective repositioning of soft tissue and allow for the best possible natural results.
- Opening the neck through a submental incision may be required for the effective management of deep neck problems.

INTRODUCTION

The group of patients who are seeking facial rejuvenation is globally becoming increasingly multicultural.[1] Ethnicity and race are both social constructs, concepts related to human ancestry, with race tending to categorize certain distinctive objective physical characteristics, whilst ethnicity tends to be more broadly used to categorize one's self-identity across language, culture, and religion.[2] The terms "race" and "ethnicity" are often interchangeably used by researchers and collapsed into a single dimension, or "ethnorace."[3] The "gold standard" for racial/ethnic assessment is self-report,[4] which means "people are who they say they are."

Differences in facial skeleton morphology across races were comprehensively studied by Farcas[5] and others.[6,7] However, there have been no published anatomic studies detailing differences in soft tissues, such as facial fat compartments or muscles across ethnic groups.[8] In addition, there is a paucity of information regarding facial aging across ethnicities.[9–14]

Historically, at a time when many surgeons came from a certain ethnic and cultural background with certain taught normative standards, many patients were transformed to reflect European standards of beauty, influenced by the neoclassical canons. These "canons," introduced by the ancient Greeks, are now thankfully recognized as incapable of being inclusive of all ethnic beauty.[6,7,15–19] Sadly, some patients do desire some form of transformation, perhaps to avoid ethnic or racial prejudice. There has also been a noted shift toward ethnic restoration where some patients experienced a loss of identity or rejection resulting from such alterations. Most patients seek preservation of racial identity with rejuvenation, and the question then arises as to whether techniques for such preservation require any form of adaptation whatsoever.

[a] FACEISTANBUL, Istanbul, Turkey; [b] FACEISTANBUL, Private Practice, Caddebostan, Ünsal Apartmanı, Bağdat Caddesi, Vezir Sk. D: No: 4/2, 34728 Kadıköy, Istanbul, Turkey
* Corresponding author. 9 Harley Street, London, W1G 9QY, United Kingdom.
E-mail address: david@ent.org.uk

Facial Plast Surg Clin N Am 30 (2022) 489–498
https://doi.org/10.1016/j.fsc.2022.07.004

The sophisticated facial plastic surgeon must not only be a master of applied anatomy but also be able to disentangle the racial, ethnic, sociocultural, and interpersonal motives of our modern cross-cultural patient populations. Surgeons must have a clear understanding of the differences between racial preservation and transformation and be able to communicate this effectively to their patients. The approach to each patient should be individualized,[2] and the surgeon must evaluate each patient's desires rather than attempt to impose their own views on "typical" ethnic features. This may help in part to negate the surgeon's own inherent biases.

AGEING DIFFERENCES AMONG ETHNICITIES

One of the most discernible characteristics is the amount of melanin pigment, though it can vary quite dramatically within ethnic groups. Darker skin with more melanin tends to maintain its structural integrity longer than those with lighter skin and shows the effect of ultraviolet radiation and DNA damage later in life.[20] Differences between skin extend beyond pigmentation, with darker skin having more cellular layers with increased adhesions. Fibroblasts are more numerous, larger, and more active with collagen bundles more parallel to the epidermis.[9] It is for these reasons that fine rhytids are less pronounced than in lighter-skinned individuals. It has been reported that more darkly pigmented individuals retain skin properties that are younger compared with lighter-pigmented individuals.[21] The less pigmented skin seems more susceptible to photoaging and atrophies more rapidly compared with other ethnicities, and it would seem that light-pigmented Caucasian skin is aging faster and is clinically more fragile and thinner than darker skin.[13] This area of research, regarding facial skin pigmentation, ultraviolet exposure, skin thickness, and aging, needs further exploration. Although it has been reported by authors that the facial skin of African Americans, Mestizos,[22] and East Asians[23] tends to be thicker and heavier,[24] this is controversial, as it has also been published that there is no significant difference in non-sun-exposed skin thickness between white and black women.[25,26] Furthermore, most authors who have studied the ultrastructural features of black skin agree that there are no structural differences other than the "packaging" and the number of melanosomes.[27,28] Aging black skin has many features of aging white skin.[29]

In general, African Americans are 15 times more likely to develop incision site keloids when compared with Caucasians.[30] Asian skin seems to carry a potential for greater fibroblast response post-surgery that may be associated with prolonged erythema, pigmentation, and hypertrophic scarring along incision lines.[31] Asian patients have a threefold increased rate of hypertrophic scarring compared with Caucasians. Informed consent should cover the potential for prolonged healing with hyperpigmentation and hypertrophic or keloid scarring because of greater fibroblast activity. Some authors recommend prophylactic scar prevention with topical silicon therapy.[31] Patient selection, informed consent, meticulous skin handling, closure with tension reduction sutures, maintaining moisture during wound healing, and alternative management techniques, such as corticosteroid injection and prophylactic silicon gels may be helpful during postoperative care.[32–34]

As skin loses its elasticity and hangs, tethered in part by the retaining ligaments of the face and neck, fine wrinkles develop. Although it would be naive to apply these heuristic shortcuts to all, fine rhytids have a greater propensity to develop earlier in Caucasians than in Hispanics, African Americans, and East Asians.[21] Therefore, traditional superficial musculoaponeurotic system (SMAS) face and neck lift techniques of Caucasians can predispose more to the delayed lateral or vertical sweep phenomenon seen postoperatively with these traditional techniques. The sweep phenomenon can be resistant to correction by revision with a repeat of the traditional SMAS facelift.[35,36] The complete release of the facial retaining ligaments is necessary to correct this most unsightly phenomenon using an extended facelift technique.[36,37] Other ethnicities, particularly African Americans[20,38] and Asians,[39] see aging manifestations in deeper structures of the face that are not primarily of skin origin, such as the SMAS, mimetic muscles, and adipose tissue. While soft tissue envelope laxity is less common in Asians than in Caucasians, the first signs of facial aging are often in the periorbital region[38] and midface, with the prominence of the nasolabial folds and a double-convexity of the midface[20] developing. Therefore, facelift techniques that include the true release of the anchoring ligaments of the midface allow for the adequate repositioning of lax tissues and are ideal for these patients to obtain a harmonious and natural result.[36,40]

Initial signs of aging in Indians were noted much earlier than Caucasians.[10] The most common esthetic concerns are malar volume loss and jowls, followed by marionette lines, with a deep prejowl sulcus appearing earlier in Indians due to their smaller lower facial framework. Midfacial volume loss is a major cause for concern in Caucasians within their fifth decade, followed by Latin

Americans and Asian populations in their sixth decade. It is then in the sixth decade that Caucasians and Latin Americans present with perioral lines, but Asians are not especially troubled until the seventh decade.[9] While the concern over the progressive deepening of the nasolabial fold occurs in all ethnicities except African Americans by the fourth decade, concern over irregularities around the tear trough region appears in all ethnicities barring African Americans by the fifth decade. In general, people of African descent have a 10-year advantage over all other ethnicities when it comes to these regions.

Concerns regarding the aging neck across ethnicities remain largely unknown because of the paucity of publications in this regard. Darker skin is generally accepted to maintain its elasticity for longer.[21] Therefore, direct neck approaches without skin excision are a possible option for such patients, even at relatively older ages.

COMMON FEATURES OF FACIAL AGING ACROSS ALL ETHNICITIES

There is no escaping the stigma of facial aging. Despite controversy with regards to differences in skin attributable to race, overall, we are all very similar. In all ethnicities, the attenuation of the retaining ligaments with age leads to the downward displacement of the facial fat compartments. This is responsible for much of the stigma attached to age. The most noticeable changes with age occur over the mobile SMAS located in front of the fixed SMAS and anterior-inferior to the zygomatic cutaneous and masseteric cutaneous ligaments[39,41,42] **(Fig. 1)**. The descent and deflation of this midfacial soft tissue in an anterior and inferior direction contributes to jowling, loss of definition at the jawline, marionette lines, prominent nasolabial folds, and volume loss in the malar region with both ptosis and atrophy of the skin and fat. Similarly, blunting of the cervicomental angle, platysmal bands, and laxity of the skin coupled with submental fat are the main stigmas of the aged neck for all.[43] Presently, for all ethnicities, a youthful facial contour rates highly for perceived health,[44] and it is well documented and widely accepted that a volumized yet smooth face with a defined neckline and subtle demarcations between facial subunits tends to appear youthful and healthy. A slender, well-defined neck with a small amount of fat and a sharp lower mandibular border is ideal. There should be no tethering, hollowing, or pendulous regions, and therefore the elasticity of the skin envelope should be maintained in all positions and from all angles.[45,46]

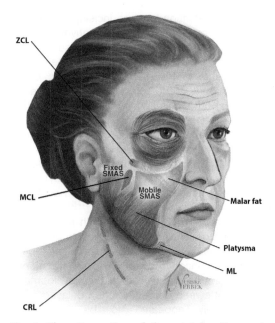

Fig. 1. The attenuation of the retaining ligaments leads to the downward displacement of the soft tissues of the face responsible for many of the stigma that occur with aging. The most prominent changes that occur with aging are anterior and inferior to the zygomatic and masseteric cutaneous ligaments (mobile SMAS). Retaining ligaments prevent the effective upward traction by suspension sutures to the SMAS of the face. Releasing of the zygomatic cutaneous ligament is important for malar repositioning, releasing of masseteric cutaneous ligaments is important for the effective correction of jowling, and releasing of mandibular ligament is important for correction of the prejowl sulcus and marionette lines. Releasing of cervical retaining ligaments is important for maximum improvement of the neck and definition of mandibular contours.

FACE AND NECKLIFT OPTIONS

The descriptive wording used to classify the variety of techniques of "face lifting" can at times seem confusing but reflects the development, heritage, and ingenuity of this surgery by passionate individuals through time.

Regarding the depth and extent of the surgical dissection, techniques can be divided into three groups. The first or "skin-only" techniques have been largely abandoned since the development of the SMAS technique by Skoog.[47] His technique allowed tension to be taken off the skin whilst also affecting changes beyond what was possible with earlier forms of facelift.

The second group is the traditional SMAS techniques of plication and imbrication.[48] Plication involves the folding over of the SMAS and its suturing into position without any incision of the

SMAS.[49] Imbrication involves incising the SMAS with a subsequent excision or alternatively a transposition, with or without a limited sub-SMAS dissection.[50] Neither technique divides the retaining ligaments of the midface (zygomatic cutaneous and masseteric cutaneous ligaments) and, therefore, both are limited in their ability to lift the midface and effect change to the nasolabial crease. The retaining ligaments of the face prevent effective traction by suspension sutures to the SMAS of the face. Inadequate or no release of the ligaments often leads to an unbalanced, unnatural appearance with an uncorrected nasolabial fold that remains despite surgery.[51–53] Attempts to improve the nasolabial folds with techniques, such as fat grafting to the malar region are more likely to result in a bizarre "overinflated" or "operated appearance." Additionally, the traditional SMAS techniques can lead to the development of a lateral sweep deformity, often delayed after what initially appeared to be successful surgery.[35,36]

The third group, or extended facelift techniques, involves the release of zygomatic cutaneous and masseteric cutaneous ligaments. SMAS dissection is advanced toward the midface along the superficial surface of the zygomaticus muscles, which allows for the repositioning of the malar fat. The correction of the nasolabial fold is only possible with the complete release of the zygomatic cutaneous ligaments, en bloc elevation of midfacial descendant tissues, and unopposed traction in a vertical vector (see **Fig. 1**). By releasing these retaining ligaments, it is then possible to reposition the midfacial soft tissue, reduce the depth of the nasolabial folds, and restore a more youthful lid–cheek junction contour without an operated appearance. Extended facelifts result in a balanced, harmonious rejuvenation of the midface, cheeks, and lower face without requiring a separate midface lift procedure.[51–53] Overall, it would therefore seem logical to restore perceived health and youth to all racial subtypes by addressing the main concerns of all ethnicities: the deepening nasolabial folds and midfacial changes.[36,37,54] However, the problem is that most facelift surgeons are hesitant to transect the retaining ligaments during a facelift because of the risk of facial nerve injury and the complex anatomy. The prezygomatic space dissection[55] (under or deep to the orbicularis oculi muscle) allows for a wide and adequate exposure of the main zygomatico-cutaneous ligament and safe release.[37,56,57] Moreover, a recent systematic review and meta-analysis showed that extended techniques while identifying and preserving the anatomy often lead to lower complication rates

than the commonly held belief that it is better to avoid vital structures by blindly working around them.[58]

The main extended facelift techniques include the deep plane,[51] the composite plane,[36] the extended SMAS,[59] and the high SMAS technique.[60] The deep plane[51] or composite techniques[52] have the advantage of elevating the flap as a single laminated unit composed of skin, malar fat, and SMAS (**Fig. 2**). This helps to preserve a robust vascular supply to the skin whilst also avoiding the unnecessary dissection of the fixed SMAS over the parotid. The composite facelift technique includes the inferior portion of the orbicularis muscle so that a stronger flap is preserved and that in turn helps to reposition the ptotic malar fat more effectively while also diminishing the nasolabial folds [40,52] (**Figs. 3** and **4**).

The neck lift is often neglected and given less attention than the face lift. Careful analysis will often reveal that for many, the main problem is not the face but the neck. A variety of different techniques have been used to improve the changes seen within the neck, but they are often tailored to the needs of the individual patient. The hallmark of a surgeon committed to his or her craft is apparent by the way in which he or she manages the aging neck.

The lateral pull of the platysma through a facelift incision is very effective in producing a tight neck. However, neck esthetics can be further improved by releasing the retaining ligaments of the neck and undertaking myotomies to the platysma

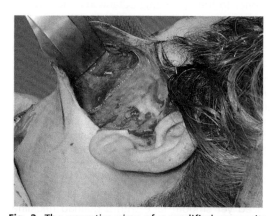

Fig. 2. The operative view of a modified composite facelift shows a wide sub-SMAS dissection with complete release of zygomatic and masseteric ligaments allowing for the effective repositioning of an "en bloc" composite flap consisting of the orbicularis oculi muscle, malar fat, SMAS (platysma), and skin. ZMM indicates the zygomaticus major muscle, and the dotted white line shows the sub-SMAS (deep plane) entry point.

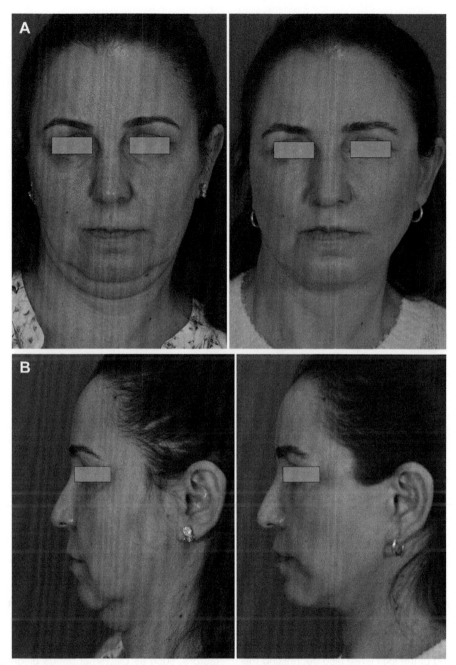

Fig. 3. (*A*) and (*B*) Preoperative (*left*) and 1-year postoperative (*right*) photos of a patient who underwent a modified composite facelift with extended neck dissection, and deep neck work through submental incision.

muscle so that it can be redraped more effectively over the deep neck structures.[61,62] The cervical retaining ligaments secure the platysma to the sternocleidomastoid muscle and prevent the mobilization and redraping of the platysma during neck and facelift surgery (see **Fig. 1**). Extending the subplatysmal dissection 4 to 5 cm inferior to the mandible allows for the safe release of the cervical retaining ligaments.[54,56,59,61,63] Adding a horizontal myotomy below the mandible can facilitate a dual vector suspension that improves the cervical contouring and enhances the jawline rejuvenation whilst avoiding blunting of the jawline contour.[56,63] In most cases, a wide subcutaneous undermining should be considered to allow for adequate redistribution, redraping, and

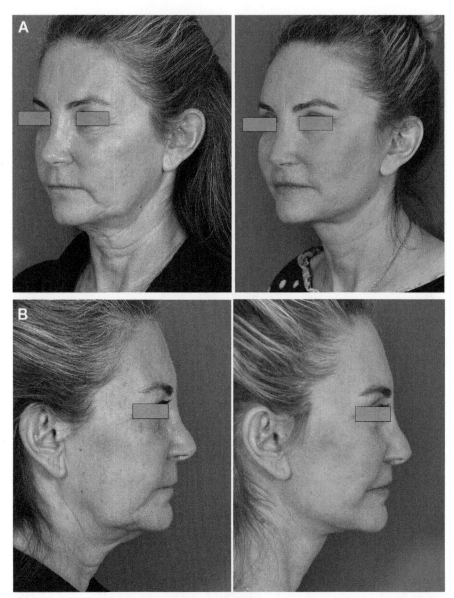

Fig. 4. (*A*) and (*B*) Preoperative (*left*) and 6 months postoperative (*right*) photos of a patient underwent modified composite facelift with extended neck dissection, and deep neck work through submental incision.

repositioning of the skin while also decreasing the horizontal neck lines due to tight adhesions between the skin and deep structures. This helps to effectively eliminate the stigma of aging in the neck.[64–66] Although closed liposuction of subcutaneous fat is one of the most common techniques applied to improve neck contours, excess removal can lead to potential problems, such as unpredictable tethering, scaring, and skeletonization of the neck. Trimming of fat with scissors under direct vision through a submental incision helps to reduce such problems.[64,66,67] Besides, there are almost always some additional contributing factors, such as platysmal bands or dehiscence, subplatysmal fat, prominent digastric muscles, and submandibular glands that can interfere with exceptional neck rejuvenation.[64–67] Opening the neck through a submental incision allows for the management of such deep neck problems and can avoid the requirement of further revision neck rejuvenation surgery. Midline platysmaplasty techniques are often required for optimum results where there is excess or redundancy of the platysma muscle.[65,68] Subplatysmal fat can be a significant covert contributor to neck aging.[67,69] It is vital that removal of subplatysmal fat is undertaken

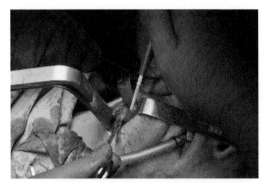

Fig. 5. Operative photo shows partial reduction of the anterior belly of digastric muscle with a cutting cautery to improve the deep neck profile.

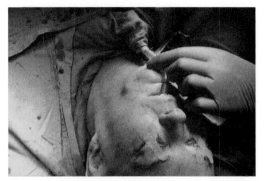

Fig. 7. Image shows subcutaneous release of the mandibular retaining ligament (ML) through the submental incision. This approach protects the marginal mandibular nerve from injury and allows the effective release of the ML helping to address the prejowl sulcus and marionette lines.

carefully and artistically, as excess removal between the two digastric bellies can lead to an esthetically unattractive "dug out" neck contour when performed without a reduction in the digastric muscle volume.[66,67] Additional contributing factors to the obtuse neck are the prominent anterior bellies of the digastric muscles and hypertrophied submandibular glands. Partial removal of these deep neck structures assists in achieving a more desirable smooth and slender neck contour[64,66,67,70,71] (**Figs. 5** and **6**). In an otherwise well-executed neck lift, the avoidance of deep neck work is often complained about by patients and can be seen by the well-trained eye in postoperative photos. As an ancillary procedure, the release of the mandibular retaining ligaments (**Fig. 7**) effectively addresses the prejowl sulcus and marionette lines and is often a prerequisite. Due to its proximity to the marginal branch of the facial nerve, a subcutaneous plane through a midline submental incision is preferred as a safe approach.[72] Additional procedures may be beneficial for the management of mid-facial volume either through restoration by autologous fat transfer or reduction with buccal fat pad removal in some ethnicities/individuals.

SUMMARY

There is an ongoing shift in the utilization of cosmetic procedures across ethnicities. Durable, natural-looking rejuvenation is not attainable unless the changes seen in aging are addressed effectively and harmoniously in all ethnicities. Although rejuvenation surgery shares common goals, the surgeon must consider each patient's individual motivations for surgery whilst also being aware of their own unconscious biases when it comes to ethnicity, aging, and beauty. Informing the patient on the limitations of the surgeries because of their specific condition, offering more aggressive techniques with additional maneuvers, and providing realistic expectations are extremely important. Face and neck lift techniques that involve the complete release of retaining ligaments of the midface and neck will facilitate the effective repositioning of soft tissue and allow for the best possible natural results. Inadequate release of these ligamentous attachments may lead to an unbalanced, unnatural appearance and may potentially result in the lateral sweep phenomenon. Additional maneuvers, such as fat injection, platysmaplasty, subplatysmal fat removal, partial resection of digastric muscles or submandibular glands may be required to provide long-term patient satisfaction.

DISCLOSURE

The authors have nothing to disclose.

REFERENCES

1. Prendergast TI, Ong'uti SK, Ortega G, et al. Differential trends in racial preferences for cosmetic surgery procedures. Am Surg 2011;77(8):1081–5.

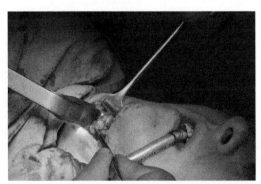

Fig. 6. The operative view showing hypertrophied right submandibular gland before its partial removal.

Available at: https://www.ncbi.nlm.nih.gov/pubmed/21944528.

2. Sturm-O'Brien AK, Brissett AEA, Brissett AE. Ethnic trends in facial plastic surgery. Facial Plast Surg 2010;26(2):69–74.

3. Kaufman JS, Cooper RS. Commentary: considerations for use of racial/ethnic classification in etiologic research. Am J Epidemiol 2001;154(4):291–8.

4. Kaufman JS. How inconsistencies in racial classification demystify the race construct in public health statistics. Epidemiology 1999;10(2):101–3.

5. Farkas LG, Katic MJ, Forrest CR, et al. International anthropometric study of facial morphology in various ethnic groups/races. J Craniofac Surg 2005;16(4):615–46.

6. Le TT, Farkas LG, Ngim RCK, et al. Proportionality in Asian and North American Caucasian faces using neoclassical facial canons as criteria. Aesthet Plast Surg 2002;26(1):64–9.

7. Porter JP. The Average African American Male Face. Arch Facial Plast Surg 2004. https://doi.org/10.1001/archfaci.6.2.78.

8. Larrabee Wayne F Jr, Scott Bevans. Surgical Anatomy of the Face: Evaluating Racial Diferences. In: Cobo R, editor. Ethnic Considerations in facial plastic surgery. Thieme Medical Publishers; 2016. p. 9–19.

9. Alexis AF, Grimes P, Boyd C, et al. Racial and Ethnic Differences in Self-Assessed Facial Aging in Women: Results From a Multinational Study. Dermatol Surg 2019;45(12):1635–48.

10. Shome D, Vadera S, Khare S, et al. Aging and the Indian face: an analytical study of aging in the Asian Indian face. Surg Glob Open 2020;8(3):e2580. Available at: https://www.ncbi.nlm.nih.gov/pmc/articles/pmc7253281/.

11. Rossi AM, Eviatar J, Green JB, et al. Signs of Facial Aging in Men in a Diverse, Multinational Study: Timing and Preventive Behaviors. Dermatol Surg 2017;43(Suppl 2):S210–20.

12. Nouveau-Richard S, Yang Z, Mac-Mary S, et al. Skin ageing: a comparison between Chinese and European populations. A pilot study. J Dermatol Sci 2005;40(3):187–93.

13. Vashi NA, de Castro Maymone MB, Kundu RV. Aging differences in ethnic skin. J Clin Aesthet Dermatol 2016;9(1):31–8. Available at: https://www.ncbi.nlm.nih.gov/pubmed/26962390.

14. Talakoub L, Wesley NO. Differences in perceptions of beauty and cosmetic procedures performed in ethnic patients. Semin Cutan Med Surg 2009;28(2):115–29.

15. Karaca Saygili O, Cinar S, Gulcen B, et al. The validity of eight neoclassical facial canons in the Turkish adults. Folia Morphol 2016;75(4):512–7.

16. Bozkir MG, Karakas P, Oguz O. Vertical and horizontal neoclassical facial canons in Turkish young adults. Surg Radiol Anat 2004;26(3):212–9.

17. Pavlic A, Trinajstic Zrinski M, Katic V, et al. Neoclassical canons of facial beauty: Do we see the deviations? J Craniomaxillofac Surg 2017;45(5):741–7.

18. Burusapat C, Lekdaeng P. What Is the Most Beautiful Facial Proportion in the 21st Century? Comparative Study among Miss Universe, Miss Universe Thailand, Neoclassical Canons, and Facial Golden Ratios. Plast Reconstr Surg Glob Open 2019;7(2):e2044.

19. Jayaratne YSN, Deutsch CK, McGrath CPJ, et al. Are neoclassical canons valid for southern Chinese faces? PLoS One 2012;7(12):e52593.

20. Brissett AE, Naylor MC. The aging African-American face. Facial Plast Surg 2010;26(2):154–63.

21. Rawlings AV. Ethnic skin types: are there differences in skin structure and function? Int J Cosmet Sci 2006;28(2):79–93.

22. Cobo R, García CA. Aesthetic surgery for the Mestizo/Hispanic patient: special considerations. Facial Plast Surg 2010;26(2):164–73.

23. Shirakabe Y. The Oriental aging face: an evaluation of a decade of experience with the triangular SMAS flap technique in facelifting. Aesthet Plast Surg 1988;12(1):25–32.

24. Lam SM. Aesthetic strategies for the aging Asian face. Facial Plast Surg Clin North Am 2007;15(3):283–91.

25. Whitmore SE, Sago NJ. Caliper-measured skin thickness is similar in white and black women. J Am Acad Dermatol 2000;42(1 Pt 1):76–9.

26. Richards GM, Oresajo CO, Halder RM. Structure and function of ethnic skin and hair. Dermatol Clin 2003;21(4):595–600.

27. Montagna W, Carlisle K. The architecture of black and white facial skin. J Am Acad Dermatol 1991;24(6 Pt 1):929–37.

28. Szabó G, Gerald AB, Pathak MA, et al. Racial differences in the fate of melanosomes in human epidermis. Nature 1969;222(5198):1081–2.

29. Herzberg AJ, Dinehart SM. Chronologic aging in black skin. Am J Dermatopathol 1989;11(4):319–28.

30. Ogawa R. Keloid and Hypertrophic Scars Are the Result of Chronic Inflammation in the Reticular Dermis. Int J Mol Sci 2017;18(3). https://doi.org/10.3390/ijms18030606.

31. Kim S, Choi TH, Liu W, et al. Update on scar management: guidelines for treating Asian patients. Plast Reconstr Surg 2013;132(6):1580–9.

32. Brissett AE, Sherris DA. Scar contractures, hypertrophic scars, and keloids. Facial Plast Surg 2001;17(4):263–72.

33. Niessen FB, Spauwen PHM, Schalkwijk J, et al. On the Nature of Hypertrophic Scars and Keloids: A Review.

Plast Reconstr Surg 1999;104(5):1435. Available at: https://journals.lww.com/plasreconsurg/Citation/1999/10000/On_the_Nature_of_Hypertrophic_Scars_and_Keloids__A.31.aspx. Accessed January 9, 2022.

34. Sherris DA, Larrabee WF, Murakami CS. Management of scar contractures, hypertrophic scars, and keloids. Otolaryngol Clin North Am 1995;28(5):1057–68. Available at: https://www.ncbi.nlm.nih.gov/pubmed/8559572.

35. Jacono AA, Malone MH. Vertical Sweep Deformity After Face-lift. JAMA Facial Plast Surg 2017;19(2):155–6.

36. Hamra ST. Building the composite face lift: A personal odyssey. Plast Reconstr Surg 2016;138(1):85–96.

37. Cakmak O, Emre IE. Surgical Anatomy for Extended Facelift Techniques. Facial Plast Surg 2020;36(3):309–16.

38. Odunze M, Rosenberg DS, Few JW. Periorbital aging and ethnic considerations: a focus on the lateral canthal complex. Plast Reconstr Surg 2008;121(3):1002–8.

39. Wong CH, Hsieh MKH, Mendelson B. Asian Face Lift with the Composite Face Lift Technique. Plast Reconstr Surg 2022;149(1):59–69.

40. Cakmak O, Emre IE, Özücer B. Surgical approach to the thick nasolabial folds, jowls and heavy neck-how to approach and suspend the facial ligaments. Facial Plast Surg 2018;34(1):59–65.

41. Alghoul M, Codner MA. Retaining Ligaments of the FaceReview of Anatomy and Clinical Applications. Aesthet Surg J 2013;33(6):769–82. Available at: https://academic.oup.com/asj/article-abstract/33/6/769/198068.

42. Furnas DW. The retaining ligaments of the cheek. Plast Reconstr Surg 1989;83(1):11–6.

43. Smith RM, Papel ID. Difficult Necks and Unresolved Problems in Neck Rejuvenation. Clin Plast Surg 2018;45(4):611–22.

44. Bater KL, Ishii LE, Papel ID, et al. Association Between Facial Rejuvenation and Observer Ratings of Youth, Attractiveness, Success, and Health. JAMA Facial Plast Surg 2017. https://doi.org/10.1001/jamafacial.2017.0126.

45. Emre İE, Ö Çakmak. Ageing face, an overview–aetiology, assessment and management. Otorhinolaryngologist Volüme 2013;6.

46. Hodgkinson D. Total Neck Rejuvenation, Harnessing the Platysma in the Lower Neck and Décolletage. Aesthet Plast Surg 2021. https://doi.org/10.1007/s00266-020-02068-4.

47. Skoog TG. Plastic surgery: New methods and Refinements. WB Saunders Company; 1974.

48. Webster RC, Smith RC, Papsidero MJ, et al. Comparison of SMAS plication with SMAS imbrication in face lifting. Laryngoscope 1982;92(8 Pt 1):901–12.

Available at: https://www.ncbi.nlm.nih.gov/pubmed/7047959.

49. Tonnard P, Verpaele A, Monstrey S, et al. Minimal access cranial suspension lift: a modified S-lift. Plast Reconstr Surg 2002;109(6):2074–86.

50. Baker DC. Lateral SMASectomy. Plast Reconstr Surg 1997;100(2):509–13.

51. Hamra ST. The deep-plane rhytidectomy. Plast Reconstr Surg 1990;86(1):53–61 [discussion: 62-3]. https://www.ncbi.nlm.nih.gov/pubmed/2359803.

52. Hamra ST. Composite rhytidectomy. Plast Reconstr Surg 1992;90(1):1–13.

53. Stuzin JM, Baker TJ, Gordon HL. The relationship of the superficial and deep facial fascias: relevance to rhytidectomy and aging. Plast Reconstr Surg 1992;89(3):441–9 [discussion 450-1]. Available at: https://www.ncbi.nlm.nih.gov/pubmed/1741467.

54. Marten TJ. High SMAS facelift: combined single flap lifting of the jawline, cheek, and midface. Clin Plast Surg 2008;35(4):569–603. vi-vii.

55. Mendelson BC. Anatomic study of the retaining ligaments of the face and applications for facial rejuvenation. Aesthet Plast Surg 2013;37(3):513–5.

56. Cakmak O, Özücer B, Aktekin M, et al. Modified Composite-Flap Facelift Combined With Finger-Assisted Malar Elevation (FAME): A Cadaver Study. Aesthet Surg J 2018;38(12):1269–79.

57. Cakmak O. Clarification Regarding the Modified Finger-Assisted Malar Elevation (FAME) Technique. Aesthet Surg J 2019;39(5):NP161–2.

58. Jacono AA, Alemi AS, Russell JL. A Meta-Analysis of Complication Rates Among Different SMAS Facelift Techniques. Aesthet Surg J 2019;39(9):927–42.

59. Stuzin JM, Baker TJ, Gordon HL, et al. Extended Smas Dissection as an Approach to Midface Rejuvenation. Clin Plast Surg 1995;22(2):295–311.

60. Barton FE. The "High SMAS" Face Lift Technique. Aesthet Surg J 2002;22(5):481–7.

61. Mustoe TA, Rawlani V, Zimmerman H. Modified deep plane rhytidectomy with a lateral approach to the neck: an alternative to submental incision and dissection. Plast Reconstr Surg 2011;127(1):357–70.

62. Jacono AA, Talei B. Vertical neck lifting. Facial Plast Surg Clin North Am 2014;22(2):285–316.

63. Jacono AA, Bryant LM, Ahmedli NN. A Novel Extended Deep Plane Facelift Technique for Jawline Rejuvenation and Volumization. Aesthet Surg J 2019;39(12):1265–81.

64. Marten TJ, Feldman JJ, Connell BF, et al. Treatment of the full obtuse neck. Aesthet Surg J 2005;25(4):387–97.

65. Feldman JJ. Neck lift my way: an update. Plast Reconstr Surg 2014;134(6):1173–83.

66. Marten T, Elyassnia D. Neck Lift: Defining Anatomic Problems and Choosing Appropriate Treatment Strategies. Clin Plast Surg 2018;45(4):455–84.

67. Auersvald A, Auersvald LA, Oscar Uebel C. Subplatysmal Necklift: A Retrospective Analysis of 504 Patients. Aesthet Surg J 2017;37(1):1–11.

68. Feldman JJ. Corset platysmaplasty. Plast Reconstr Surg 1990;85(3):333–43.

69. Marten TJ, Elyassnia D. 67 - Neck Lift. In: Farhadieh RD, Bulstrode NW, Mehrara BJ, et al, editors. Plastic surgery - Principles and Practice. Elsevier; 2022. p. 1041–81. https://doi.org/10.1016/B978-0-323-65381-7.00067-8.

70. Connell BF, Shamoun JM. The significance of digastric muscle contouring for rejuvenation of the submental area of the face. Plast Reconstr Surg 1997;99(6):1586–90. Available at: https://www.ncbi.nlm.nih.gov/pubmed/9145126.

71. Mendelson BC, Tutino R. Submandibular Gland Reduction in Aesthetic Surgery of the Neck: Review of 112 Consecutive Cases. Plast Reconstr Surg 2015;136(3):463–71.

72. Jacono A, Bryant LM. Extended Deep Plane Facelift: Incorporating Facial Retaining Ligament Release and Composite Flap Shifts to Maximize Midface, Jawline and Neck Rejuvenation. Clin Plast Surg 2018;45(4):527–54.

Skeletal Contouring Techniques in the Ethnic Patient

Kofi Boahene, MD

KEYWORDS

- Malarplasty • Mandibuloplasty • Zygomaticomaxillary complex • Ostectomy • Corticectomy

KEY POINTS

- The zygomaticomaxillary complex and the mandible are key bones of beauty amenable to safe esthetic contouring in cases of excess.
- Key principles that guide reduction malarplasty and mandibuloplasty are centered around preserving function, with an eye on esthetic goals.
- Preserving bone-to-bone contact is of paramount importance in malar reduction to avoid nonunion and associated challenges.

INTRODUCTION

Across the globe, irrespective of race or ethnicity, facial beauty is a neurobiological interpretation of a visual intake. What the eye beholds as beautiful is a visual perception of a composition of light reflected off the face and evaluated for proportions, symmetry, and averageness. This visual composition is then judged within the context of cultural inputs, familiarity, and imprinting.[1–5] What an observer perceives as a surface reflection is greatly defined by the underlying facial structure that shapes the overlying soft tissues. When the facial skeleton places lights and shadows in the right places, the result is a harmonious visual image. The importance of facial skeleton in determining facial form, function, and esthetics has been of interest to many professionals including forensic anthropologists, dentists, sculptors, and surgeons. In this article, we will review key facial bones of beauty and how their excesses can be surgically modified to enhance facial beauty.

THE BONES OF BEAUTY: FORM, FUNCTION, AND INFLUENCE ON BEAUTY

The facial bones that serve as a foundation for the soft tissues of the midface and lower face are the primary "bones of beauty."[6–8] They determine the facial proportions, projection, symmetry, contour, and how light casts defining highlights and shadows on the face.

In the midface, the zygomaticomaxillary complex (ZMC) is the major determinant of facial form as it supports the eye, the nose, upper dentition, and muscles of facial muscles expression. The maxilla, together with the articulating zygomatic bone, in their anterior–posterior projection and horizontal expanse, is critical in the overall appearance of the face on frontal view and has consequential functional implications (**Fig. 1**). The development of the zygomaticomaxillary complex is linked to dentoalveolar development and is often the focus of early orthodontic manipulation to prevent later deformities.

There are elaborate and detailed cephalometric parameters for objectively evaluating the dimension of the maxilla and zygomatic bones relative to the skull base.[9] Although these metrics are important to craniofacial surgeons, they are not easily understood by laypersons whose primary interest is esthetics. Simplified terminologies and metrics that describe the face as flat, prominent, wide, or long are helpful when discussing treatment options with patients. Depending on the anterior–posterior projection of the zygomaticofacial complex, the

Otolaryngology head and neck surgery, Johns Hopkins, 601 N caroline st, 6th floor JHOC, Baltimore, MD 21050, USA
E-mail address: dboahen1@jhmi.edu

Facial Plast Surg Clin N Am 30 (2022) 499–506
https://doi.org/10.1016/j.fsc.2022.08.001
1064-7406/22/

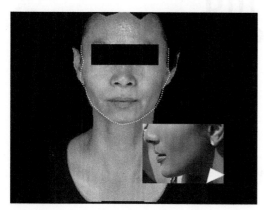

Fig. 1. Facial contour and shadows. White triangle showing gonial shadow.

midfacial shapes can be esthetically described as concave, convex, or neutral. The prominence of each of the above types of facial profiles among various ethnic groups, sexes, and their esthetic implications have been extensively addressed in the orthognathic and plastic surgery literature. Midfacial advancement surgery with orthognathic manipulation, Leforte osteotomies or midfacial augmentation with onlay implants will not be addressed here. Rather, we will focus on excesses in midfacial width that is best addressed with reduction contouring surgery.

Zygoma Reduction (Malarplasty)

Much has been written about midfacial augmentation with implants when the zygomaticomaxillary complex is retrusive or hypoplastic. However, the reduction of zygomaticomaxillary complex is less widespread outside Asia. Among Asians, zygoma reduction surgery is popular because their culture often elevates the slender oval facial contour over other shapes. Although malar bone reduction is performed to a lesser extent among non-Asians, the technique for malar bone excess is similar.

Conceptually, malarplasty is like surgically introducing some of the changes seen following unrepaired ZMC fractures where the malar complex becomes inwardly rotated. In cosmetic malarplasty, a controlled narrowing of the ZMC is performed for esthetic goals. Ideal candidates for malar bone reduction have appropriate dentoalveolar relationship but a wide midface or anterior projection because of malar bone prominence. In these patients, reducing the malar bone is performed primarily to achieve a smoother and more harmonious facial esthetic lines. Although the deformity is usually bilateral, unilateral malar hypertrophy and treatment occurs. When dentoalveolar abnormalities are present, a more

comprehensive restructuring with Le forte type osteotomies and maxillomandibular alignment is preferred.

Computed tomographic (CT) scans with 3-dimension constructs are useful when analyzing the shape of the malar bone to determine the most projecting aspects that are targets for reduction. There are several tools that can aid in presurgical planning, including patient-specific surgical guides, CT scan with morphing algorithms, and surgical models.[10]

Several important principles should guide surgical planning and ostectomies.

First, stability of the malar complex postreduction is paramount. This requires bone-to-bone contact. Second, the line of masticatory forces along the lateral buttress should not be disturbed. Third, substantial bone-to-bone step-off should be avoided. Fourth, attachment of the masseter muscle must be maintained. Fifth, the orbicularis oculi and zygomatic branches of the facial nerve are at risk and must be protected. Sixth, avoiding violation of the maxillary sinus is desirable. Seventh, the temporomandibular joint is sacred and should be protected.

The malar bone is exposed through a sublabial incision similar to the approach for repairing ZMC fractures. Care is taken to preserve an ample mucosal strip to facilitate a watertight closure. The opening to the parotid duct should be identified and avoided. Dissection to expose the underlying bones should be subperiosteal. For proper orientation the lateral maxillary buttress, zygomaticomaxillary suture line, zygomatic body, lateral orbital rim, and infraorbital foramen should be visualized. Next, preplanned malar bone reduction is executed factoring in asymmetry and the degree of narrowing desired.

Surgery to reduce lateral projection of the malar bones has evolved over time with techniques that include shaving, osteotomy with setback, and ostectomies with fixation. Among Asian patients where dramatic malar contouring is desirable, different permutations of an L-shaped malar ostectomy with fixation has become popular.[11–16] The above outlined principles should serve as a valuable guide regardless on one's preferred technique.

In the high L-malar osteotomy, a beveled arch osteotomy is planned at the narrowest point of zygomatic arch, approximately 8 mm anterior to the articular tubercle of zygomatic root. A parallel ostectomy is planned to remove a strip of bone 3 to 5 mm depending on the degree of narrowing desire. The ostectomy is placed medial to the most projecting aspect of the malar eminence. A second osteotomy through the most concave point of the zygomatic frontal process was planned. The lateral orbital rim and maxillary buttress are preserved (**Fig. 2**).

The zygomatic arch can be exposed through a small incision around the temporal hair tuft. Care should be taken to stay behind the course of frontal branch of the facial nerve to avoid brow paralysis. Once expose and osteotomy through the arch is performed with a bevel to allow bone-to-bone contact once the mobilized zygoma has been advanced to narrow the malar width and zygomatic arch projection.[17] Low-profile plates are then placed for stable fixation. Bone step-offs at the malar should be contoured down. The surgical site is irrigated out, and the mucosal access incision closed in a watertight manner. Patients may be given a tapered dose of steroid and encouraged to ice the cheeks to minimize swelling. A soft diet for 2 weeks allows early bone healing before exerting chewing forces on the arch by thew masseter muscle.

In cases where minimal-to-moderate reduction is desired, we have found incremental shaving and reduction of the malar bones still valuable. With this method, the area of desired bone reduction is outlined with a side cutting burr or ultrasonic bone scalpel down to the targeted depth. Next, the ultrasonic bone dissected is used to evenly reduce the malar bone down to the desired depth. Although this approach may be slow and painstaking, it is safe and effective and avoids any issues associated with complete bone interruption such as instability, malunion, nonunion, and masticatory problems.

Common complications following malarplasty include bone nonunion with associated instability and masticatory challenges. Additional compilations include numbness, asymmetry, and failure to achieve desired goals.

Mandibular Contouring

The esthetics of lower face is influenced primarily by the shape, size, orientation, and projection of the mandible.[18] The effect of the mandible on facial esthetics is most notable on profile and three-quarter views, revealing the facial height, the jaw line, chin projection, and the transition of the face to the neck (see **Fig. 1**). Although the side profile is often ignored in traditional facial beauty analysis, it is as relevant as the frontal view because it reveals proportions of the upper, middle, and lower face and is important is assessing dentoalveolar health and balance. Features that may look appropriate on frontal view may be completely out of balance on profile and three-quarter views and distort the observers' composite facial beauty assessment and one's esthetic appeal. There are racial and ethnic differences in skeletal profile parameters that should be considered when analyzing the facial skeleton for potential esthetic manipulation. In addition, beauty standards among Eastern, African, and Western cultures differ and should be considered when counseling patients.

The height of the mandible is determined by the length and orientation of the mandibular ramus and its length and projection by the mandibular body (**Fig. 3**). The mandibular ramus grows relatively vertical downward, and its height is relevant for generating the necessary moment arm for masticatory biting forces.[19] Men generally have more height to their ramus compared with women. Women with a longer mandibular rami will have more masculine features. This strong jaw loon in women, although undesirable in Eastern cultures, is commonly seen among Western runway models. Jaws that generate strong biting forces are also associated with larger masticatory muscles. Masseter muscle hypertrophy, in such cases, can add to the width of the lower face hence the use of Botulinum toxin injection for lower facial narrowing.[20]

The angle between the mandibular ramus and body at the gonion defines the jaw angle or gonial angle. The gonial angle is a sexually dimorphic trait

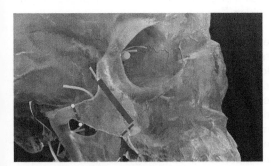

Fig. 2. Parallel malar osteotomy.

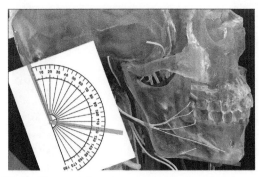

Fig. 3. The gonial angle.

with men and women having different characteristic angles. For men, the gonial angle is around 128° and for women, around 126°.[21,22] Although the difference in gonial angle between men and women is not substantial, differences in ramus height is more distinguishing between the two sexes.[21,22] There is an inverse correlation between the ramus height and gonial angle. The shorter the ramus, the less horizontal the mandible body grows resulting is an obtuse gonial angle with associated dentoalveolar challenges. An obtuse gonial angle is associated with lower facial rounding and lack of definition.

The Gonial Shadow

An important yet often overlooked facial esthetic feature in the gonial shadow. The gonial shadow is a reflection of a defined mandibular ramus in both anterior posterior and lateral projections. It focuses the observer's eye to the highlights of the jaw because it transitions to the neck (see **Fig. 1**). In the profile or three-quarter view, the gonial shadow is more visible in youth and thin necks but becomes blunted with aging and weight gain. Restoring the neckline and recreating the gonial shadow is a desirable outcome in neck lift surgery.

The width of the lower face determines whether one has a squarish or oval looking face on front view (**Fig. 4**). The width of the lower face is determined primarily by the distance between the mandibular gonions, the bigonial width. Although a wide bigonial width is traditionally accepted as a desirable male feature, this is often seen among female models. In general, prominent and wide bigonial widths are common reasons women patients seek jaw contouring surgery for a more feminine look.

Mandibular and Gonial Angle Contouring

When evaluating the mandible for lower facial reshaping, categorizing the mandibular excess into 3 subgroups is helpful in surgical planning: (1) A posterior inferiorly positioned gonion (a closed gonial angle) in women will benefit from gonial angle widening using a V-line ostectomy; (2) A wide bigonial distance with an appropriate gonial angle should be treated with a tangential or outer cortex reduction only; and (3) When a posteroinferiorly positioned gonion is associated with a wide bigonial distance, both a curved V-line ostectomy and outer corticotomy is indicated[23] (**Fig. 5**).

Just as with malar bone reduction, certain principles are helpful when planning and executing mandibular reduction surgeries.

First, function should not be compromised for esthetics. For example, overreduction of the ramus height can alter attachment and function of the masticator muscles, alter chewing forces with adverse dietary implications.

Second, the inferior alveolar nerve and marginal branch of the facial nerve are at risk and their injury can be devastating to patients. Third, the inferior alveolar nerve course within the target area for mandibular reduction and should be protected.

Presurgical planning with various tools available to surgeons is helpful in precisely targeting areas for contouring, ensuring symmetric outcomes, and minimizing operating time. When available, 3-D printed patient-specific skulls are helpful. Sterile templates can be taken off the skull models and used as intraoperative surgical guides.[24]

Under general anesthesia, the mandibular is exposed through a gingivobuccal incision that extends from a midpoint between the upper and lower molars down the lateral crest of the external oblique ridge and ending near the ipsilateral canine. The mental nerve fibers at the level of the canine are superficial and can be injured when making this mucosal incision. A cuff of tissue, when preserved around the mental nerve can act as a protective barrier against inadvertent injury. To facilitate closure, the mucosal cuff should be

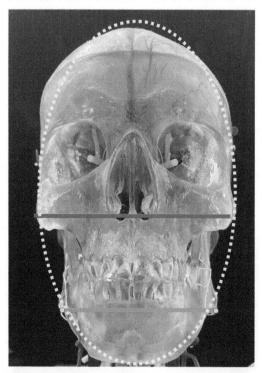

Fig. 4. Bones of beauty: intermallar (blue line) and intergonial widths (green line).

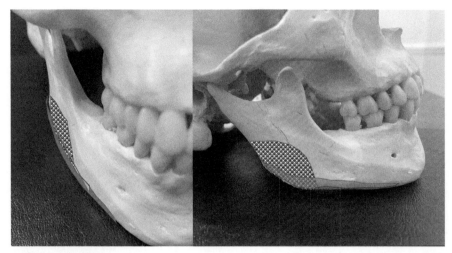

Fig. 5. Lower facial reshaping.

generous to facilitate watertight closure. As an alternative, a periapical incision may be used.

Dissection to expose the mandibular body and ramus is subperiosteal. Appropriate soft tissue retractors are then placed to broadly expose the targeted areas as well as protect the surrounding soft tissue. It should be noted that the facial artery can be injured with this procedure resulting in a bloody field and more complications.

Once the targeted area is exposed, the preplanned template is placed and the outline clearly marked to guide symmetric ostectomies. Using a reciprocating saw and osteotomes, corticectomy of the lateral aspect of the mandibular ramus followed by "V" ostectomy of the mandibular base can then be performed. The V-line ostectomy of the gonion and inferior border of the mandible is challenging without the right instrument. An angled oscillating saw and transcutaneous perforating osteotomies are helpful in this regard.

We have also found the ultrasonic bone scalpel a useful tool for mandibular contouring given its safety profile around delicate soft tissues when exposure is limited.

Appreciating of the intraosseous course of the inferior alveolar nerve on preoperative scans is a prerequisite for performing mandibular osteotomies.[25,26] The course of the inferior alveolar nerve varies in the general population and cannot be reliably predicted based on surface anatomy only. Ascertaining the course in individual patients using radiographs is therefore advisable.

As noted earlier, hypertrophic masseter muscles are often associated with higher biting forces seen in patient with long mandibular ramus height. In such patients, resecting a layer of masseter muscle may be complimentary. When considered, masseter muscle resection should be performed on the deeper aspect of the muscle to avoid injury to the overlying facial nerve.

Complications associated with mandibular angle reshaping include asymmetry, masseter muscle malposition, and inadequate reduction. These risks can be minimized with careful planning guided by the previously outlined principles. When well executed, the results from mandibular contouring can be dramatically positive.

Case Sample

A 25-year-old Caucasian woman interested in feminizing of the lower face. She had no dentoalveolar challenges.

Examination revealed moderate thickness facial skin, grossly symmetric facial halves. Frontal view analysis showed appropriate midfacial width and wide intergonial width resulting in a lack of facial definition and a squarish lower face. Profile and three-quarter analysis showed a long ramus height, an acute gonial angle, the presence of a gonial shadow, retropositioned chin and a defined jaw line. At rest and with clenching, a moderately hypertrophic masseter muscle was noted.

A recommendation for gonial angle contouring was given. Through a transoral approach, a gonial angle reshaping with cortical ramus and body reduction was performed. Additional buccal fat reduction was performed for further definition. **Fig. 6** shows outcome at 3 months after operative visit.

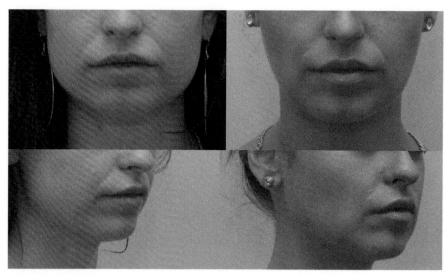

Fig. 6. Gonial angle contouring 3-month postoperative result.

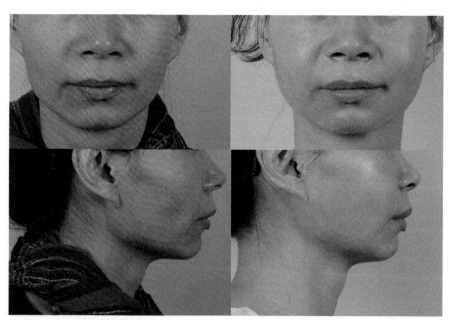

Fig. 7. A 1-cm retromandibular incision, cortical reduction, and gonial angle reshaping 3-month postoperative result.

Case 2

A 28-year-old woman presented with concerns for a wide midface with prominent cheekbones as well as prominent jaw angles. Examination show wide intermalar width, prominent zygomatic arches, prominent gonial angles, and a moderately wide intergonial distance.

Through a sublabial approach, the malar bone and zygomatic arches were contoured and reduced in projection using a shave down technique with an ultrasonic bone dissector. Through a 1-cm retromandibular incision, cortical reduction and gonial angle reshaping was performed. **Fig. 7** shows results at 3 months.

CLINICS CARE POINTS

- During the preoperative discussions, the potential for cheek and chin numbness, even temporary, and possible need for revision should be emphasized.

- A trial of Botox injection into the masseter muscles, when hypertrophic, should be considered before proceeding with bone reduction when the lower facial width is primarily on frontal view and the gonial angle is satisfactory. Patients get a sense of what their result can be and are psychologically better prepared for the surgical outcome.

REFERENCES

1. Skov M, Nadal M. The nature of beauty: behavior, cognition, and neurobiology. Ann N Y Acad Sci 2021;1488(1):44–55.
2. Zhang W, Lai S, He X, Zhao X, Lai S. Neural correlates for aesthetic appraisal of pictograph and its referent: An fMRI study. Behav Brain Res 2016; 305:229–38.
3. Little AC, Jones BC, DeBruine LM. Facial attractiveness: evolutionary based research. Philos Trans R Soc Lond B Biol Sci 2011;366(1571): 1638–59.
4. Rhodes G. The evolutionary psychology of facial beauty. Annu Rev Psychol 2006;57:199–226.
5. Coetzee V, Greeff JM, Stephen ID, Perrett DI. Cross-cultural agreement in facial attractiveness preferences: the role of ethnicity and gender. PLoS One 2014;9(7).
6. Jefferson Y. Skeletal types: key to unraveling the mystery of facial beauty and its biologic significance. J Gen Orthod 1996;7(2):7–25.
7. Chung Seungil, Park Sanghoon. The Aesthetic Midface Analysis: Diagnosis and Surgical Planning. Facial Bone Contouring Surg Springer Singapore 2017;135–43.
8. Woo HK, Ajmera DH, Singh P, Li KY, Bornstein MM, Tse KL, Yang Y, Gu M. Evaluation of the relationship between malar projection and lower facial convexity in terms of perceived attractiveness in 3-dimensional reconstructed images. Head Face Med 2020;16(1):8.
9. Sarver D, Jacobson RS. The aesthetic dentofacial analysis. Clin Plast Surg 2007;34(3):369.
10. Kang SH, Tak HJ, Kim HJ, Lee SH. Reduction malarplasty using a simulated surgical guide for asymmetric/prominent zygoma. Head Face Med 2022; 18(1):11.
11. Lee Tae Sung. Standardization of surgical techniques used in facial bone contouring. J Plast Reconstr Aesthet Surg 2015;68(12):1694–700.
12. Baek SM, Chung YD, Kim SS. Reduction malarplasty. Plast Reconstr Surg 1991;88:53–61.
13. Cho BC. Reduction malarplasty using osteotomy and repositioning of the malar complex: clinical review and comparison of two techniques. J Craniofac Surg 2003;14:383–92.
14. Mahatumarat C, Rojvachiranonda N. Reduction malarplasty without incision, 2003 external incision: a simple technique. Aesthet Plast Surg 2003;27: 167–71.
15. Sumiya N, Ito Y, Ozumi K. Reduction malarplasty. Plast Reconstr Surg 2004;113:1497–9.
16. Yang X, Mu X, Yu Z, et al. Compared study of Asian reduction malarplasty: wedge-section osteotomy versus conventional procedures. J Craniofac Surg 2009;20:1856–61.
17. Lee Tae Sung, Park Sanghoon. Advantages of a Beveled Osteotomy on the Zygomatic Arch During Reduction Malarplasty. J Craniofac Surg 2017; 28(7):1847–8.
18. Avelar LET, Corradi LM. Mandible: evaluation of its morphology, aging process and sexual dimorphism for aesthetic treatment purpose. J Dermat Cosmetol 2021;5(3):42–6.
19. Said AV, Takaki PB, Vieira MM and et al Relationship between maximum bite force and the gonial angle in crossbite Dent, Dent Oral Craniofac Res, 2017. Volume 3(5): 1-5
20. Shome D, Khare S, Kapoor R. Efficacy of Botulinum Toxin in Treating Asian Indian Patients with Masseter Hypertrophy: A 4-Year Follow-Up Study. Plast Reconstr Surg 2019;144(3).
21. Balaji SM, Balaji P. Square Face Correction by Gonial Angle and Masseter Reduction. Ann Maxillofac Surg 2020;10(1):66–72.
22. Taleb NSA, Beshlawy ME. Mandibular Ramus and Gonial Angle Measurements as Predictors of Sex and Age in an Egyptian Population Sample: A

Digital Panoramic Study. J Forensic Res 2015;6: 308.

23. Li J, Hsu Y, Khadka A, Hu J, Wang Q, Wang D. Surgical designs and techniques for mandibular contouring based on categorisation of square face with low gonial angle in orientals. J Plast Reconstr Aesthet Surg 2012;65(1).

24. Yi CR, Choi JW. Three-Dimension-Printed Surgical Guide for Accurate and Safe Mandibuloplasty in Patients With Prominent Mandibular Angles. J Craniofac Surg 2019;30(7):1979–81.

25. Kim YH, Jeon KJ, Lee C, Choi YJ, Jung HI, Han SS. Analysis of the mandibular canal course using unsupervised machine learning algorithm. PLoS One 2021;16(11).

26. Liu T, Xia B, Gu Z. Inferior alveolar canal course: a radiographic study. Clin Oral Implants Res 2009; 20(11):1212–8.

Rhinoplasty Considerations in the Ethnic Patient Using a Case-Based Approach
The Patient of African Descent

Sean P. McKee, MD[a], Kofi Boahene, MD[b], Anthony E. Brissett, MD[c],*

KEYWORDS

- African rhinoplasty • Rhinoplasty • Ethnicity • Race

KEY POINTS

- For patients who have recently undergone filler placement, it is prudent to allow 6 to 12 months to elapse, depending on the type of filler used, before proceeding with rhinoplasty to allow the product time to naturally resorb.
- The surgical principles of rhinoplasty, including exposure techniques, cartilage grafting, suture modification, and soft tissue modification can be effectively executed by open structure and endonasal techniques
- With growing rates of cosmetic procedures, including rhinoplasty, among patients of African descent, it is important to understand anatomic characteristics in the context of the desired nasal features in addition while appreciating the importance of racial/ethnic preservation.

INTRODUCTION

The African continent comprises more than 50 countries with a population of roughly 1.4 billion people.[1] Beyond the borders of the continent, the African diaspora has a population of 140 million with Brazil, Colombia, the United States, Dominican Republic, and Haiti being among the most populated countries.[2] The diversity of the diaspora reveals an equally diverse array of anatomic variability within the face and nose, and this is reflected by significant variability of facial and more specifically nasal features. Despite the differences in nasal features that may exist between racial or ethnic groups of African descent, a common principle exists among patients seeking rhinoplasty; a desire to improve upon balance, symmetry, and harmony that works to complement one's overall facial appearance.

As the interest for rhinoplasties continues to increase among patients of African descent and the expectation that postsurgical rhinoplasty results will focus upon outcomes that emphasize cultural and racial preservation, it is imperative that the rhinoplasty surgeon appreciate anatomic characteristic, global concepts of beauty, as well as racial/ethnic facial and nasal features.[3]

There are no financial conflicts of interest to disclose.
[a] Department of Otorhinolaryngology - Head and Neck Surgery, McGovern Medical School of the University of Texas Health Science Center at Houston, 6431 Fannin Street, MSB 5.036, Houston, TX 77030, USA;
[b] Otolaryngology Head and Neck Surgery, Department of Otolaryngology Head and Neck Surgery, Division of Facial Plastic and Reconstructive Surgery, The Johns Hopkins University School of Medicine, Johns Hopkins Outpatient Center, 601 N. Caroline Street, 6th Floor, Baltimore, MD 21287, USA; [c] Department Otolaryngology/ Head and Neck Surgery, Division of Facial Plastic and Reconstructive Surgery, Houston Methodist Hospital, Weill Cornell College of Medicine, Smith Tower, 6550 Fannin Street, Suite 1703, Houston, TX 77030, USA
* Corresponding author.
E-mail address: aebrissett@houstonmethodist.org

Facial Plast Surg Clin N Am 30 (2022) 507–511
https://doi.org/10.1016/j.fsc.2022.08.002
1064-7406/22/© 2022 Elsevier Inc. All rights reserved.

Successful rhinoplasty outcomes will therefore depend on executing desired modifications using modern rhinoplasty techniques in the context of ethnically sensitive preferences among patients of African descent. Herein, 2 rhinoplasty cases involving patients of African descent are presented. One of these highlights the correction of a dorsal contour irregularity and an amorphous and ptotic tip with a widened alar base, addressed through an open approach. The second case focuses on improving nasal tip definition through an endonasal approach.

CASE PRESENTATION
Patient 1

A 30-year-old West African woman presented for discussion with regard to improving the esthetic appearance of her nose. In general, she was unhappy with the overall nasal appearance. Her primary concerns included her profile, notably an underprojected dorsum, a dorsal contour irregularity magnified by moderate depression of the middle third, along with an underrotated and underprojected nasal tip with an acute nasal labial angle and excess columellar show. From the frontal view (Fig. 1A), she was unhappy with the width of her bony and alar base along with her possessing an amorphous, poorly defined and ptotic tip. From a functional standpoint, she described left-sided nasal obstruction. The patient was referred to the authors' office by a plastic surgeon who had completed injections of hyaluronic acid into the nasal dorsum and tip 3 months before the initial consultation at the authors' office.

Upon examination (see Fig. 1A), on frontal view, she has a dorsal contour irregularity with a slight dorsal hump along the upper third of her nose and mild saddling along the middle third of her nose. The lower third of her nose is characterized by a wide and amorphous nasal tip that is underprojected, ptotic, and underrotated with an acute nasolabial angle with increased columellar show. The basal view (Fig. 1B) reveals both increased base width and alar flaring and a shortened columella. To address her concerns, the authors discussed performing a functional septoplasty and turbinate reduction as well as an open structure rhinoplasty addressing her dorsal contour irregularities in addition to improving upon the appearance of the nasal tip and nasal base.

Surgical Procedure

The procedure was performed under general anesthesia with endotracheal tube intubation. The functional septoplasty was performed first through a hemitransfixion incision followed by a turbinate reduction. Posterior, dorsal, and caudal chondrotomies were made to resect the deviated portion of the septum with great care to preserve the dorsal and caudal struts. The interseptal space was then reconstituted with AlloDerm and closed with a continuous quilting suture. The inferior turbinates were then outfractured and reduced using radiofrequency ablation.

Once the functional aspects of the procedure were completed, an open rhinoplasty approach was used to address the esthetic concerns. A transcolumellar and marginal incisions were

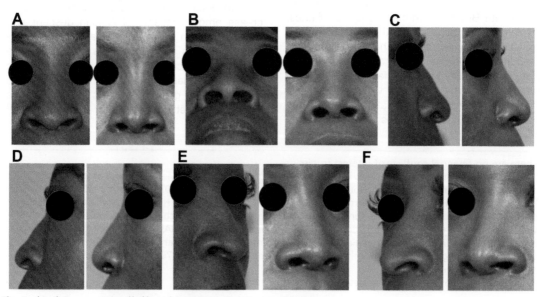

Fig. 1. (A–F) Preoperative (left) and postoperative images (right).

completed, and the soft tissue envelope was elevated off the lower lateral cartilages, upper lateral cartilages, and nasal dorsum. Remnants of the previous injected hyaluronic acid filler could be visualized in the subcutaneous tissue along the tip and dorsum. The vestibular lining was released from the lateral crura on both the left and right sides and a 3-mm lateral crural steal was performed. Tip refinement was then accomplished with both interdomal and intradomal sutures. A columellar strut graft was then placed between the medial crura from the anterior nasal spine to the nasal tip. The osseous component of the dorsal hump was rasped and the cartilaginous portion was shaved sharply. A crushed cartilage onlay graft extending from the depressed middle third of the nasal dorsum down to the lower lateral cartilages was placed and secured with a 5-0 polydioxanone (PDS) suture. A layer of AlloDerm was placed over the cartilage graft along the entire length of dorsum, and a crushed cartilaginous plumping graft was placed along the nasolabial angle. Cephalic trim of the lower lateral cartilage was performed while preserving 9 mm of lateral crus. A septocolumellar suture was placed, the soft tissue envelope was redraped, and the transcolumellar and marginal incisions were closed. A 3-mm ala base excision was performed along the nasal sill on both sides. Nasal skin taping, internal silastic splints, and an external nasal splint were applied.

Surgical Outcome

Postoperative photographs were taken 1 year after the surgery (**Fig. 1**). The contour along the nasal dorsum is greatly improved through the reduction of the bony and cartilaginous dorsum hump and augmentation of the middle third. The nasal tip demonstrates increased rotation and projection with refinement of the nasal tip and tip-defining points. She also has a narrowed alar base and reduced flare, softened nasolabial angles, and an elongated columella while maintaining symmetric nasal sills.

Discussion

The first consideration in this case is the timing for performing the procedure. The patient initially presented after having undergone hyaluronic acid filler injection to the nasal tip and dorsum. Her previous treatment with hyaluronic acid fillers raises the question of the optimal time to operate. The authors ultimately elected to delay proceeding with surgery until 6 months after the hyaluronic acid injection was performed to allow time for the material to resorb naturally.[4,5] This delay not only

provided a more accurate assessment of her natural nasal features but also mitigated the effect that hyaluronidase injection may have on the soft tissue envelope.

The esthetic concerns of this patient were then primarily addressed through modifications to the dorsal contour, nasal tip, and lower lateral cartilages. An improved dorsal contour can be appreciated in the profile view in **Fig. 1**C, D.

Additional nasal features addressed included an underrotated nasal tip, increased alar base width, and an underprojected anterior nasal spine, commonly observed nasal features in patients of African descent seeking rhinoplasties.[2] In this case, modifications to tip rotation and projection were accomplished through a combination of techniques, including a lateral crural steal, suture modifications, and cartilage grafting. These maneuvers provided nasal tip rotation, projection, and refinement. A cartilage plumping graft was placed in a pocket overlying the anterior nasal spine softening the nasolabial angle.

CASE PRESENTATION
Case 2

A 28-year-old African American female presented with a desire to seek improvement in her nasal appearance. Her primary concerns were the appearance of her nasal tip, nostrils, and dorsal width. She requested improvement in tip projection and definition as well as narrowing of the alar base. On examination, the nasal skin was intermediately thick and sebaceous. From the frontal view (**Fig. 2**A), her tip was broad, amorphous, and lacking in definition with increased alar flare and increased alar base width. From a lateral view (**Fig. 2**B), the nasal tip is underprojected and shows a relative dorsal hump accentuated by her decreased tip projection. A prominent alar crease can also be appreciated from both lateral views (**Fig. 2**C, D). In addition, the anterior nasal spine is diminutive resulting in an acute nasolabial angle. Her nasal bridge is also broad.

Surgical Procedure

The procedure was performed under general anesthesia with endotracheal tube intubation and was executed by an endonasal approach. The desired areas of light reflection and contrasting shadows were drawn into place. Using calipers the width of her Cupid's bow was measured and set to guide the positioning of the newly desired tip defining points. The septum was accessed and cartilage was harvested by a hemitransfixion incision while marginal incisions allowed access

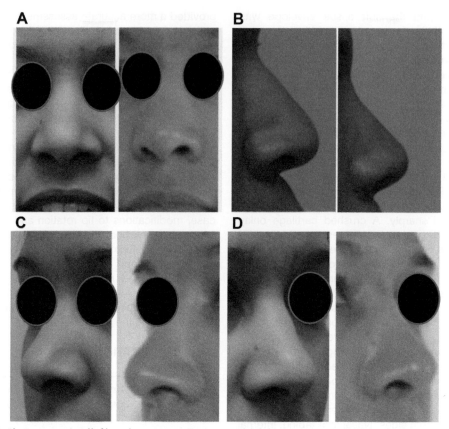

Fig. 2. (A–D): Preoperative (left) and postoperative images (right).

to the medial and lateral crura, soft tissue envelope, and the premaxilla.

Through the marginal incisions, the soft tissue envelope was elevated from the upper and lower lateral cartilages. The skin enveloped was then selectively debulked down to the dermal plexus. Next, using a 1-mm osteotome, guiding continuous paramedian osteotomies were performed to help narrow the wide dorsum. To accentuate the dorsum, low lateral perforated osteotomies were then performed using a transcutaneous technique. The nasal bones were then contoured to create desired sidewall shadows.

An end-to-side septal extension graft was then sutured into place. The vestibular lining was released off the lateral crura. The lateral and intermediate crura were then delivered through the marginal incisions. Suture modification of the intermediate crura was completed with intradoma and interdomal sutures followed by lateral crural spanning sutures and lateral crural strut grafts to strengthen and flatten their relatively convex contour. The restructured lateral crural cartilage were transposed more caudally into newly dissected pockets and stabilized with draw sutures through the alar crease. Tip projection was created by

suture modification and fortified by supporting the medial crura on the septal extension graft in a tongue-and-groove style. Alar rim grafts were deployed through the marginal incisions into a precise pocket along the alar rim. Once modification of the cartilaginous structures was completed, attention was then turned to the soft tissue envelope. The soft tissue envelope was redraped and all access incisions closed.

The nostrils and alar base were further reduced and reshaped through 4-mm intrasill excisions. The resulting defect was closed with 4-0 PDS sutures and 5-0 fast absorbing sutures. Finely diced cartilage packed into a 1-mL syringe was then injected into a precisely dissected dorsal pocket mainly to accentuate dorsal light reflection. Internal and external nasal dressing were applied and removed on postoperative day 7.

Surgical Outcome

Postoperative photographs were taken at 1 year following surgery (see **Fig. 2**A–D). The projection and definition of the nasal tip and refinement to nasal appearance in general are greatly improved. The combination of cartilage grafting, suture techniques, and modification of the soft tissue envelope allow for improvement in the overall appearance. Alar flare is diminished by increasing tip projection along with the placement of alar rim grafts, and the increased alar base width is minimized by performing alar base excisions.

Discussion

This case reflects the ability to provide significant modifications to the nasal tip and dorsum in a patient with thick skin through an endonasal approach. The use of a septal extension graft reflects the need to provide tip support while subtly augmenting the premaxilla. In addition, despite the structural changes that allow for increased tip projection and definition such as cartilage grafting and suture techniques, the soft tissue envelope frequently needs to be addressed. In this case debulking the soft tissue envelope overlying the nasal tip and performing alar base excisions allowed for refinement to the overall appearance.

REFERENCES

1. Available at: https://worldpopulationreview.com/country-rankings/countries-in-africa. Accessed July 24, 2022.
2. Available at: https://www.yukonyouth.com/the-african-diaspora-what-is-it/. Accessed July 30, 2022.
3. O'Connor K, Brissett AE. The changing face of america. Otolaryngol Clin North Am 2020;53(2):299–308. Epub 2020 Feb 11. PMID: 32057407.
4. Boahene KDO. Management of the nasal tip, nasal base, and soft tissue envelope in patients of african descent. Otolaryngol Clin North Am 2020;53(2):309–17. Epub 2020 Feb 11. PMID: 32057406.
5. Kim JE, Sykes JM. Hyaluronic acid fillers: history and overview. Facial Plast Surg 2011;27(6):523–8. Epub 2011 Dec 28. PMID: 22205525.

Rhinoplasty Considerations in the Ethnic Patient Using a Case-Based Approach: The Latino Patient

Roxana Cobo, MD

KEYWORDS

- Latino rhinoplasty • Mestizo rhinoplasty • Thick skin rhinoplasty • Mesorrhine noses
- Hybrid rhinoplasty

KEY POINTS

- Latino patients are also known as mestizo or Hispanic patients. Owing to the different migration patterns today, Latino patients are considered mixed race patients.
- Latino or mestizo patients tend to have poor osteocartilaginous frameworks and nasal tips with poor rotation and projection. It is not uncommon to find patients with small humps or pseudohumps
- In patients with mesorrhine noses and small cartilaginous humps, surface cartilaginous preservation techniques are being used conserving the cartilaginous middle third of the nose intact.
- Today, a hybrid approach is used with Latino patients. Preservation and structural techniques are used in combination to obtain consistent results. Tissue is preserved, remodeled, and structured when necessary. All techniques are performed using sutures, grafts, and powered instrumentation techniques.

INTRODUCTION

Latino is usually a term that is used interchangeably with mestizo or Hispanic, and basically means patients who are coming from Latin American countries. Owing to the different migration patterns in Latin America over the years, Latino or mestizo patients are a combination of races, mainly white, African origin, and native Indians. Because of this racial mixture, it becomes important to be able to perform an adequate anatomic diagnosis in each patient and plan surgery depending on the patient's individual findings.[1]

Generally speaking, Latino patients tend to have weak bony and cartilaginous frameworks. The skin-soft tissue envelope (S-STE) tends to be thicker and tips are usually flimsy and bulbous with poor projection and rotation. It is common to find retrusive caudal septums, and availability of septal cartilage is limited, so surgery must be planned carefully.[2] In the cases where septal cartilage is not enough for the grafting needs of the patient, other harvesting options include conchal ear cartilage and costal cartilage.

In this article 2 representative cases are presented: a mestizo patient with a small hump, wide dorsum, and bulbous undefined nasal tip and a patient with a relatively flat dorsum, and a bulbous, wide undefined nasal tip with poor projection and rotation.

CASE STUDY/PRESENTATION

Case 1: Mestizo patient undergoing primary rhinoplasty. Small osteocartilaginous hump and bulbous undefined asymmetric nasal tip.

Case Presentation

A 21-year-old patient was seen with complaints of nasal obstruction due to allergies, and dislike for the shape of her nose. The patient had a small osteocartilaginous hump with a relatively weak

Department of Otorhinolaryngology, Private Practice Facial Plastic Surgery, Clinica Imbanaco, Carrera 38A #5A-100, Consultorio 222 Torre A, Cali, Colombia
E-mail address: rcobo@imbanaco.com.co

Facial Plast Surg Clin N Am 30 (2022) 513–520
https://doi.org/10.1016/j.fsc.2022.07.005
1064-7406/22/© 2022 Elsevier Inc. All rights reserved.

underlying skeleton. Her nasal tip was asymmetric, with wide, bulbous alar cartilages with poor projection and rotation. The caudal edge of the septal cartilage was retrusive and deviated to the left creating tip asymmetry. The nasal spine was small, the nasolabial angle acute, the feet of the medial crura short, and when the patient smiled, the nasal tip would plunge downward (**Fig. 1**).

Computer imaging with simulation was performed. The patient insisted she wanted a natural result that showed better projection, rotation, and definition without looking operated. What bothered her the most was the "bump" of her dorsum on the lateral view and the fact that her nasal tip looked "round and big" and when she smiled it went down. It was agreed that the dorsal hump would be lowered, the nasal bones remodeled and narrowed, and the tip refined trying to improve rotation and projection.

Surgical Procedure

The procedure was performed under general anesthesia. An open rhinoplasty approach was used where an inverted V-shaped transcolumellar incision was connected to bilateral marginal incisions. Dissection was carried out in a subdermal plane up to the supratip region leaving the superficial musculoaponeurotic system (SMAS) attached to the cartilaginous structures of the nasal tip. A flap was created elevating the SMAS en bloc with the intercrural, interdomal, and Pitanguy ligaments in a subperichondrial plane off the medial crura, dome area, and lateral crura up to the supratip area, thus creating a superiorly pediculated SMAS-ligament flap. The nasal tip and cartilaginous middle third of the nose were dissected in a subperichondrial plane, and a wide dissection of the nasal bones was performed

in a subperiosteal plane. Using an intercrural approach, the caudal edge of the nasal septum was exposed. Bilateral mucoperichondrial septal flaps were elevated in a subperichondrial plane exposing the cartilaginous and bony components of the nasal septum.

Using powered instrumentation (cylindrical cutting burs and diamond burs), the bony cap of the nasal bones was removed exposing a small cartilaginous hump. Bony irregularities were evened out. With this maneuver a bony hump was converted to a small cartilaginous hump. The cartilaginous hump was then treated using a cartilaginous pushdown technique. A subdorsal or intermediate rectangular strip (Tetris approach) was performed and a 3-mm strip was resected starting at a point where the upper lateral cartilages meet the dorsal portion of the nasal septum and extended posteriorly toward the subdorsal area of the cartilaginous dorsum. Release of the lateral keystone area was performed, and the small cartilaginous hump was pushed down resulting in a straight dorsum. Dorsal work was completed with medial and lateral osteotomies to narrow the dorsum. Internally at the level of the septum, the subdorsal strip was sutured to the remaining septum with 4-0 polydioxanone (PDS) sutures fixing it in place. Once the subdorsal strip was stabilized, cartilage was harvested for grafts preserving an inverted L of 15 mm of cartilage dorsally and caudally. The deviation at the caudal edge of the septum was corrected and the strip secured to the nasal spine with a 4-0 PDS suture fixing it securely in the midline.

The nasal tip was approached using structural techniques. An overlapping septal extension graft (OSEG) was placed on the right side of the caudal edge of the nasal septum, and stabilized on the contralateral side with a rectangular bolster graft (**Fig. 2**). The alar cartilages were sutured to the OSEG using lateral crural tensioning techniques

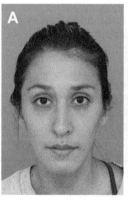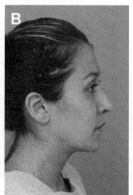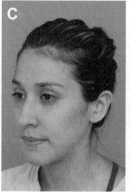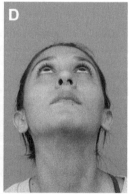

Fig. 1. (*A–D*) Preoperative images of mestizo patient showing a small osteocartilaginous hump; bulbous, undefined and asymmetric nasal tip; and a weak underlying osteocartilaginous framework.

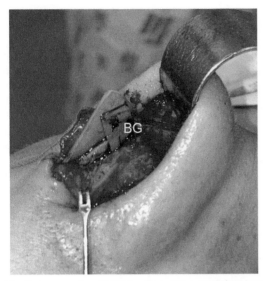

Fig. 2. Image of an OSEG in place. It is a straight piece of cartilage that is carved according to patient's needs and placed overlapping the caudal edge of the nasal septum and sutured in place. To create additional stability, a contralateral rectangular piece of cartilage is sutured in place stabilizing the graft to the caudal end of the septum (bolster graft- BG). These grafts can be fashioned from septal cartilage, conchal cartilage, or rib cartilage.

thus defining rotation and projection of the nasal tip.[3] The width of the lateral crus of the alar cartilages was reduced using a lateral crural turn in flap.[4,5] On the right side the lateral crus was repositioned in a more symmetric fashion previous placement of a lateral crural strut graft. Additional refinement techniques of the nasal tip were performed with oblique domal sutures, dome aligning sutures, and lateral crural spanning sutures. Final refinement of nasal tip area was achieved injecting a combination of finely diced cartilage (FDC) with cartilage paste (CP) and covering all tip work with the superiorly pediculated SMAS flap. The FDC and CP were used to fill in concavities in the supratip area and increase refinement in the nasal tip area over the domes. Before closing, the SMAS flap was pulled down covering the nasal tip area and sutured in place; this created a nice supratip break and helped camouflage work done in the nasal tip (**Fig. 3**).

Postoperative Outcome

The 1-year postoperative result is shown. The patient has a nice straight dorsal line with a small supratip break. There is marked improvement in the rotation, projection, and definition of the nasal tip. On the frontal view the dorsal tip esthetic lines

look narrower and the nasal tip has more definition and refinement (**Fig. 4**).

Discussion

Latin or mestizo patients have diverse nasal characteristics. Patients frequently have a modest osteocartilaginous skeleton, and surgery must be planned carefully. Harvesting options must be planned and executed precisely because the amount of cartilage available to harvest from the septum will be limited. The combination of powered instrumentation and cartilage preservation techniques to treat small osteocartilaginous humps has become a very important tool because in this way the middle third of the nose is preserved and grafts are mainly used to structure the nasal tip. Most preservation approaches that are used by the author for this type of patients are surface preservation techniques (remodeling of bony cap, resection of bony cap) or subdorsal approaches (Tetris, subdorsal Z-flap). These techniques leave enough cartilage available for harvesting once the L strut is reconstituted leaving at least 1 cm of cartilage dorsally and 1 to 1.5 cm caudally.[6–9]

Today, we are using almost exclusively septal extension grafts to define tip position. In primary patients, cartilage is harvested from the patient's nasal septum. and it is usually enough to be able to design an adequate SEG, a contralateral bolster graft, and any additional structural grafts for the nasal tip (lateral crural strut grafts or articulated alar rim grafts). Because projection is very important in most mestizo nasal tips, the graft is placed overlapping the patient's caudal septum and further stabilized using a contralateral bolster graft. Once the pedestal is stabilized, and the amount of tip projection defined, tip refinement is performed. Today most techniques are aimed at structuring and straightening the lateral crus of the alar cartilages; this can be done with tensioning techniques or placement of grafts. The final objective is a tip that looks more defined, less bulbous, but that will not lose support over time.[1]

Final refinement techniques of the nasal tip are done with grafts, sutures, or replacement of ligament structures of the nose. Small pieces of cartilage that are left over after grafts are carved are finely diced and/or scraped to create FDC paste. This cartilage paste is placed using a cartilage injector or a 1-mL tuberculine syringe in areas that need to be evened out or filled in or in areas that need more definition like the dome area in the nasal tip.

The superiorly pediculated SMAS flap is a flap that is used in patients who have normal skin

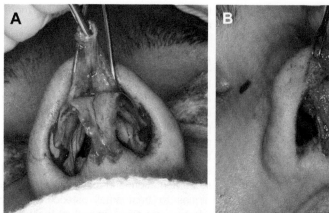
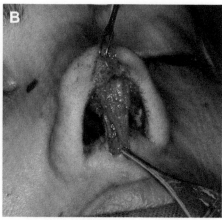

Fig. 3. (*A*) Image of the superior pediculated SMAS flap. The flap is created elevating the SMAS and the ligament structures of the nose in one block up to the supratip area (*B*). At the end of surgery the SMAS flap is lowered covering the nasal tip area. This flap serves 2 purposes: to eliminate dead space formation in supratip area and to camouflage nasal tip area.

thickness or thin skin. The flap is created when the skin flap of the open rhinoplasty approach is created. A skin flap (epidermis and dermis) is elevated over the nasal tip leaving the SMAS and all the nasal tip ligaments attached to the cartilaginous nasal structure. The SMAS flap is then created, elevating the SMAS with the intercrural, interdomal, and the Pitanguy ligaments en bloc up to the supratip area. Dissection is then continued under the flap over the bony and cartilaginous structures of the nose. At the end of surgery, the flap is pulled down over the nasal tip area and sutured back in place over the medial crura. This flap helps reduce dead space formation in the supratip area and helps re-create a nice supratip break. Additionally, it creates a nice smooth cover over the nasal tip structures hiding any irregularities.[10]

Case 2: Primary rhinoplasty with low dorsum and relatively thick S-STE.

Case Presentation

A 23-year-old female patient is seen who wants to improve the form and function of her nose. She has a long history of allergies and nasal obstruction that have not been properly treated. She feels her dorsum is "flat," dislikes her wide bulbous nasal tip, and thinks the skin over her nasal tip and ala looks overly thick. On examination, the patient has a slight septal deviation with severe turbinate hypertrophy and a retrusive caudal septum. Her dorsum is relatively flat and wide. The nasal tip shows wide, flattened alar cartilages; a retrusive caudal septum; a relatively short columella; and a wide nasal base. The S-STE is thick. A nasal computed tomographic scan was performed that showed severe inferior turbinate hypertrophy with blockage of the middle meatus and thickening of the mucosa of the maxillary sinus bilaterally.

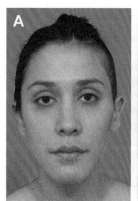
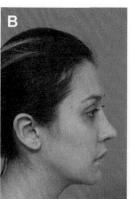
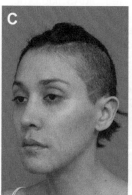
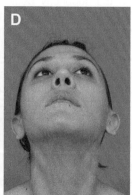

Fig. 4. (*A–D*) One-year postoperative images showing a nice straight dorsal profile with a nasal tip with improved definition, rotation, and projection.

Pictures were taken that show a relatively small nose with a small bony and cartilaginous structure. The frontal view shows a wide dorsum with a wide nasal tip. The middle third of the nose looks depressed. On the lateral and oblique views, a low dorsum is visible with an important depression in the radix and supratip area and a small pseudo-hump. The nasal tip is round and bulbous with poor projection and rotation. The nasolabial angle is acute. The base view shows a wide nasal base with flaring inverted ala (**Fig. 5**).

Computer imaging and simulation was performed. Harvesting options were discussed. It was agreed that the patient needed a surgery that would create more definition of her nasal tip. The dorsum would be augmented and narrowed, and the tip would be projected and refined. Because of the racial characteristics of the patients and the need for an important amount of cartilage for grafting, it was explained to the patient that the available septal cartilage would not be enough and other grafting options had to be explored. Rib cartilage and ear cartilage grafting options were explained to the patient with its advantages and disadvantages. It was finally decided that ear cartilage would be used for dorsal augmentation and septal cartilage would be used for structural grafts in the nasal tip area.

Operative Procedures

The surgery was performed under general anesthesia. Conchal cartilage was harvested using an anterior approach, harvesting cymba and cavum concha leaving the cartilage of the root of the helix intact. The skin flap was sutured in place placing bolster sutures in the conchal area to prevent hematoma formation. Vaseline gauzes were placed covering the concha serving as a slight pressure dressing. Next the functional aspect of the nose

was approached. An endoscopic sinus surgery was performed with endoscopic turbinectomy. Rigorous hemostasis was performed.

An open rhinoplasty approach was used where an inverted V-shaped transcolumellar incision was connected to bilateral marginal incisions. The skin flap was elevated in a subdermal plane leaving the SMAS and ligament structures attached to the cartilaginous structures of the nasal tip up to the supratip area. The SMAS covering the nasal tip area was then resected en bloc with the nasal tip ligaments (intercrural, Pitanguy) taking care not to extend dissection into the supralar groove or the middle third of the nose (**Fig. 6**). Once the SMAS was resected, the skin flap elevation was continued over the cartilaginous middle third of the nose and the bony dorsum in a subperichondrial and subperiosteal plane, exposing the bony and cartilaginous dorsum.

The septum was dissected through an intercrural approach. Bilateral anterior, inferior, and posterior tunnels were dissected. Septal cartilage was identified, deviations corrected, and cartilage harvested leaving a complete L-strut of 10 mm dorsally and caudally. A septal quilting suture was performed with 5-0 fast-absorbing vicryl closing the septal area.

Bilateral medial and lateral osteotomies were performed narrowing the lateral bony vault and preserving the middle cartilaginous vault intact. The septal cartilage that was harvested, was used to design an OSEG, bilateral articulated alar rim grafts, and a small shield graft. The OSEG was placed defining the projection of the nasal tip and stabilized further with a contralateral bolster graft. Lateral crural tensioning was performed stabilizing the newly created domes and lateral crura against the OSEG.

Once the tip and pedestal were stabilized, and the projection of the nasal tip defined, the dorsal

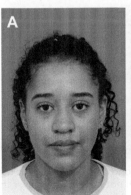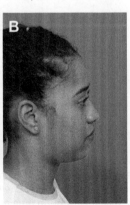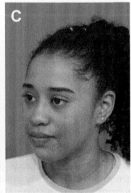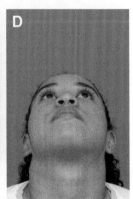

Fig. 5. (*A–D*) Preoperative photographs of a Latino patient with a nose with platyrrhine features. She has a small pseudohump with a low dorsum and wide flattened middle third of the nose. The nasal tip is bulbous with poor definition and projection, the columella is short, and the nasal base is wide.

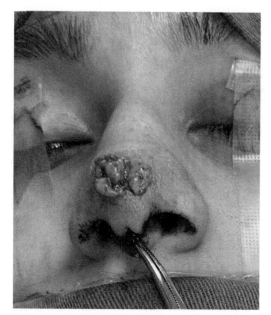

Fig. 6. Resected SMAS from nasal tip area. In patients with very thick S-STE, resecting the SMAS is a good option to thin out the S-STE and help in the nasal tip definition. The resected SMAS can then be used as a graft in other areas of the nose.

height was addressed. The conchal cartilage was finely diced and mixed with fibrin glue (Tiseel) and immediately placed in a template or mold designed from a 3-mL syringe cut lengthwise. The cartilage pieces were firmly pressed together with 2 fingertips to take out any excess glue and make sure the tiny cartilage pieces were tightly pressed together. Using this template, the diced cartilage glue graft was fashioned according to

patient's individual needs, defining length, width, and height of the graft. Once the graft was ready, it was taken out of the template and final refinements were made before being placed over the patient's dorsum. When the graft was finally shaped and ready to be inserted, the dorsal portion was covered with a thin piece of perichondrium that was glued in place covering most of the dorsal portion of the graft. The graft was then carefully inserted over the dorsum making sure the height was adequate for the patient's nasal tip position (**Fig. 7**).

Final refinement of the nasal tip was achieved with the placement of articulated alar rim grafts, and a small shield graft. The SMAS that was resected at the start of the surgery was used as a graft. One piece was placed in front of the nasal spine, and another piece was used to cover the leading edge of the shield graft over the nasal tip.

Postoperative Outcome

The patient's 9-month postoperative follow-up shows adequate dorsal augmentation with nice dorsal tip esthetic lines. Definition of her nasal tip was improved, and the nasal base looks more symmetric (**Fig. 8**).

The patient's skin was thick, oily, and acne prone. As soon as tapes were removed, the patient was placed on a skin regime with facial scrubs, skin toner, and sun block. In addition, the patient was started on a low-dose isotretinoin scheme 20 mg twice a week during 6 months. The patient was monitored periodically with hepatic function tests and birth control measures were enforced.

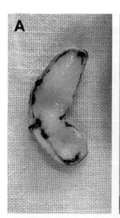
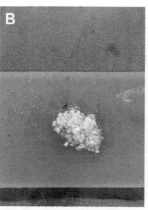
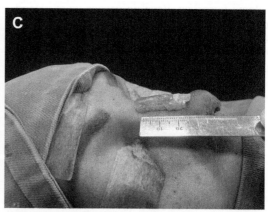

Fig. 7. Dorsal augmentation with finely diced cartilage (FDC) with fibrin glue (*A*). Conchal cartilage graft is harvested from the ear (*B*). The cartilage is diced finely making sure cartilage pieces will not be noticeable over the dorsal skin (*C*). Image of dorsal graft elaborated with FDC mixed with fibrin glue and its dorsal portion covered with perichondrium or fascia. The graft is tailored depending on the individual patient's needs. The side of the graft that is in contact with the dorsal skin is covered with perichondrium or fascia helping camouflage the finely diced cartilage pieces.

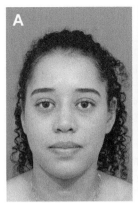 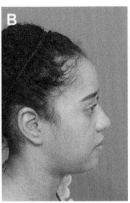 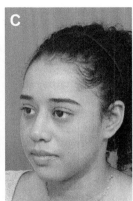 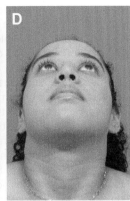

Fig. 8. (A).Nine-month postsurgical result. (B, C) Dorsum was augmented, and dorsal esthetic lines were improved. (D) The nasal tip looks more projected and refined. Nasal base is narrower, and ala configuration has been improved.

The skin evolution was favorable with complete control of her acne and sebum production.

Discussion

A percentage of mestizo patients require some form of dorsal augmentation. Many techniques can be performed to achieve this, but it is out of the scope of this article. The author for many years has been augmenting dorsums using the technique of FDC mixed with fibrin glue (diced cartilage glue graft) with excellent results.[11] This technique has a very low infection rate, and because it is not a solid piece of cartilage there is no warping. Some investigators have reported the visibility of cartilage pieces over the nasal dorsum especially in patients with thin skin.[12] To avoid this, the author for several years has covered the dorsal portion of the graft with a thin piece of perichondrium or fascia adding additional camouflage to this area of the nose. It does become important to discuss with the patient alternatives for cartilage harvesting because usually septal cartilage will not be enough to cover all of patients grafting needs especially if dorsal augmentation is going to be performed. Additional grafting sites are conchal cartilage or rib cartilage.

Skin thickness plays an important role in rhinoplasty results. For this reason it becomes important to prepare the skin for surgery and to control postsurgical skin inflammation and swelling; this can be done by prescribing cleansing agents that contain salicylic acid or benzoyl peroxide. When needed, scrubs can also be used. The objective is to remove the superficial dead skin and stimulate skin cell renewal. All patients should use sunblock, and direct sun exposure should be avoided. In all patients, a change in diet is stressed, because today we know that avoiding hyperglycemic carbohydrates, transfats, high-sugar diets, and milk and/or milk derivatives can help control acne flare-ups and inflammation.

Patients with thick skin or acne-prone skins should ideally be started on isotretinoin. Low-dose schemes are just as effective as normal dosing and have considerably less side effects (0.25 mg/kg–0.40 mg/kg). The dose can be given 2 to 3 times a week, and treatment should be continued at least during 4 to 6 months to have a permanent result on the skin. It does become imperative to make sure patients sign all pertinent consent forms and female patients guarantee they will not get pregnant during treatment. The question then becomes, when should patients be placed on isotretinoin? If patients are willing to wait for their surgery, they should be started on treatment before surgery (1–2 months) to condition skin properly. Isotretinoin is stopped 1 to 2 weeks before surgery and restarted as soon as tapes come off, 2 weeks after surgery. If patients want surgery immediately, isotretinoin is started as soon as tapes come off, which is usually 2 weeks after surgery. Today studies show that there is no reason to delay surgery when a patient is on treatment with isotretinoin and no studies confirm that the healing process will be impaired or that patients will have abnormal scarring.[13,14]

SUMMARY

When performing rhinoplasty in Latino patients 3 questions must always be answered to be able to manage patients properly: What type of underlying skeletal framework does the patient have? What type of S-STE does the patient have covering this skeleton? Will the patient's septal cartilage be enough for all the grafts that will be needed even if it is a primary rhinoplasty case? In cases in which the dorsum is low and augmentation is required, this is achieved using FDC combined with fibrin glue and covered on the dorsal side with perichondrium or fascia. These patients usually need additional cartilage that can be harvested from concha or from rib.

In those cases in which the patient has a small osteocartilaginous hump, the author today is using cartilaginous dorsal preservation techniques in an effort to preserve the middle third of the nose intact. In all cases, the tips in Latino patients are approached using a "structural preservation approach," wherein little if any tissue is resected and cartilaginous structures are reinforced using structure techniques. For all patients, the skin is treated to control postsurgical inflammation and edema with topical treatments, diet, and when necessary oral treatment with isotretinoin. The final goal of surgery is to obtain consistent results that satisfy our patients and stand the test of time.

CLINICS CARE POINTS

- Today rhinoplasty in Latino patients is done with a combination of structural and preservation techniques
- Approach to the nasal tip in Latino Patients usually requires important structural techniques to obtain long lasting rotation and projection
- When needed, dorsal augmentation is performed using grafts of finely diced cartilage mixed with fibrin glue, giving patients natural long lasting results
- Cartilaginous dorsal humps today are being treated with cartilaginous dorsal preservation techniques
- Thick acne prone skin is managed medically with low dose oral isotretinoin during 4-6 months with good results

---

DISCLOSURE

The author has nothing to disclose.

REFERENCES

1. Cobo R. Management of the mestizo nose. Otolaryngol Clin North Am 2020;53:267–82.
2. Cobo R. Rhinoplasty in latino patients. Clin Plast Surg 2016;43:237–54.
3. Davis RE. Lateral crural tensioning for refinement of the wide and underprojected nasal tip: rethinking the lateral crural steal. Facial Plast Surg Clin North Am 2015;23(1):23–53.
4. Tellioglu AT, Cimen K. Turn-in folding of the cephalic portion of the lateral crus to support the alar rim in rhinoplasty. Aesthetic Plast Surg 2007;31(3):306–10.
5. Murakami CS, Barrera JE, Most SP. Preserving structural integrity of the alar cartilage in aesthetic rhinoplasty using a cephalic turn-in flap. Arch Facial Plast Surg 2009;11(2):126–8.
6. Kosins A. Expanding indications for dorsal preservation rhinoplasty with cartilage conversion techniques. Aesthet Surg J 2021;41(Issue 2):174–84.
7. Ferreira MG, Toriumi DM. A practical classification system for dorsal preservation rhinoplasty techniques. Facial Plast Surg Aesthet Med 2021;23(Number 3):153–5.
8. Neves JC, Tagle DA, Dewes W, et al. A segmental approach in dorsal preservation rhinoplasty: the tetris concept. Facial Plast Surg Clin North Am 2021;29(1):85–99.
9. Kovacevic M, Veit J, Toriumi DM. Subdorsal Z-flap: a modification of the Cottle technique in dorsal preservation rhinoplasty. Curr Opin Otolaryngol Head Neck Surg 2021;29(4):244–51.
10. Cobo R. Superiorly Pediculated Superficial Musculoaponeurotic System Ligament Flap to Control the Supratip. JAMA Facial Plast Surg 2018;20(6):513–4.
11. Tasman AJ, Diener PA, Litschel R. The diced cartilage glue graft for nasal augmentation morphometric evidence of longevity. Facial Plast Surg 2013;15(2):86–94.
12. Tasman AJ. Dorsal augmentation-diced cartilage techniques: the diced cartilage glue graft. Facial Plast Surg 2017;33(02):179–88.
13. Cobo R, Vitery L. Isotretinoin use in thick-skinned rhinoplasty patients. Facial Plast Surg 2016;32(6):656–61.
14. Cobo R, Camacho JG, Orrego J. Integrated management of the thick-skinned rhinoplasty patient. Facial Plast Surg 2018;34(1):3–8.

Rhinoplasty Considerations in the Ethnic Patient Using a Case-Based Approach
The Middle Eastern Patient

Amani A. Obeid, MBBS, SB-ORL HNS, FACS*

KEYWORDS

- Middle East • Rhinoplasty • Platelet rich fibrin membrane • PRF

KEY POINTS

- The Middle Eastern population is very diverse, with variable nasal anatomy, skin thickness, and ideals of beauty between different regions.
- Understanding each patient specific preferences and expectations is crucial.
- A good proportion of patients in the Middle East have thick skin, proper knowledge on how to manage thick skin, medically and surgically is important in dealing with those patients.

 Video content accompanies this article at http://www.facialplastic.theclinics.com.

INTRODUCTION

The Middle East is composed of 16 countries with many different racial, ethnic, and ideological groups native to the area. Moreover, the migration of several other races to the region over centuries led to the great variation of ethnic groups in the Middle East.[1] Rhinoplasty is by far the most performed facial cosmetic surgery in the Middle East. The increased popularity of rhinoplasty among all age groups has been observed in the last decade, with social media popularity being a major attribute.[2–4]

Owing to the presence of great racial diversity in the Middle East, great variation exists in facial anatomy, nasal cartilage strength, and skin thickness.[5–7] Moreover, the ideal nasal shape varies widely between different Middle Eastern countries,

and sometimes even within different regions in the same country. Thereby the rhinoplasty surgeon should be aware of these variations and beauty ideals, as they frequently change as time goes by.

CASE ANALYSIS

The patient is a 27-year-old women with no medical comorbidities, no previous surgical history, no facial trauma, and no functional complaints. She is seeking rhinoplasty for purely cosmetic reasons. Her main concerns were the droopy tip and dorsal hump.

On examination (**Fig. 1**), she has a slight axis deviation to the left side and thin skin. A wide nasal tip that lacks definition and a wide dorsum, lack of tip support is noted on her lateral view. As a

There are no financial conflicts of interest to disclose.
Department of Otolaryngology, Head and Neck Surgery, King Saud University, King Saud University Medical City, Riyadh, Saudi Arabia
* PO Box 484, Riyadh 11411
E-mail address: amobeid@ksu.edu.sa

facialplastic.theclinics.com

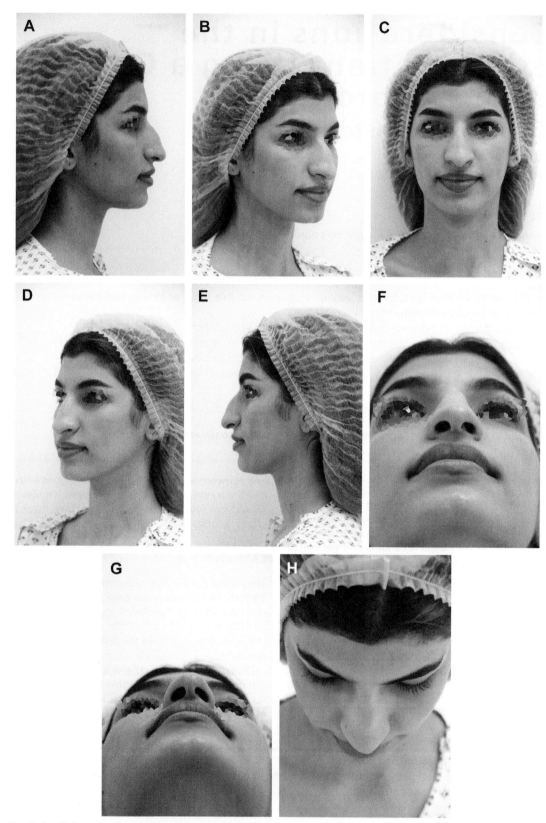

Fig. 1. (*A–H*) Preoperative patient views.

result, her tip appears to be droopy and under-projected. The increased columellar show is noted as well. She also has a dorsal hump that appears larger than its real size because of the droopy tip. Radix is in a good position and depth. It is also noted that she has an exaggerated supra-tip break, therefore reduction of the anterior septal angle should be avoided while excising the hump.

SURGICAL PLAN

The surgery was done under general anesthesia with endotracheal tube intubation. An open rhinoplasty approach was used accessing the nose through an inverted V transcolumellar incision and bilateral marginal incisions. The desired tip position was imitated using forceps to rotate the tip to better judge how much of the hump needs to be resected. The dorsum was dissected in a subperichondral/subperiosteal manner to avoid any irregularities over the dorsum. The hump was predominantly bony with a small cartilaginous component. The bony hump was excised using a 10 mm osteotome followed by a rasp to smoothen the bony edges. The 2 mm cartilaginous hump was shaved using a #11 blade, no open roof was encountered.

Septoplasty was carried on afterward, she had a septal spur on the left side, and excision of the spur along with an inferior strip of cartilage corrected her septal deviation. Attention was then shifted to her tip; conservative cephalic trimming was done leaving 8 mm of the lateral crura in place. To increase her tip rotation and projection, a septal extension graft (SEG) (**Fig. 2**) was used rather than a simple columellar strut as she needs an additional tip support. A graft from septal cartilage was used as a "clip" on the caudal septum fixing it with 5-0 polydioxanone suture (PDS) (**Fig. 3**A and B) This method has the benefit of providing an additional support as 2 pieces of cartilage are used on both sides of the septum avoiding the potential complication of the tip shifting to the side if the graft was fixed to one side. This SEG offered the desired rotation in addition to increasing projection. Domal sutures with lateral crural tensioning using 5-0 PDS were followed by dome equalizing sutures.[8,9]

Slight dorsal irregularity was palpable at the rhinion. For camouflage, a platelet-rich fibrin (PRF) membrane was made out of the patient blood and mixed with finely diced cartilage.[10] Within 5 min, the formed membrane was strong enough to be used to cover any dorsal irregularities (Video 1). Ultrafinely diced cartilage was used to fill the supra tip depression (Videos 2 and 3). Bilateral low–high osteotomies were done endonasally to narrow the bony dorsum.

Wounds were closed with 6-0 prolene®, 6-0 vicryl rapide®. Nasal taping and thermoplastic splint were applied.

OUTCOME

Postoperative photos were taken 4 mo after the surgery (see **Fig. 3**A–H). The nose is now more in harmony with her facial features. She has nice dorsal esthetic lines on the frontal view, along with a narrower, more defined tip. On the lateral view, good tip rotation is achieved with straight dorsum. No dorsal irregularities were encountered. She is happy with the results.

LESSONS LEARNT FROM THE CASE

In managing Middle Eastern patients, careful assessment of the skin's soft tissue envelope is of vital importance. In this patient with thin skin, skin irregularities are a feared complication. She also was to start isotretinoin oral treatment for body acne, which may result in further thinning of her skin, so placing an additional layer of cushioning tissue to camouflage irregularities is a good idea. Options include temporalis fascia, rectus fascia, fat grafting, and so forth. I started using PRF for over a year now and the results are comparable to temporalis fascia, but with the added advantage of sparing the patient an additional incision. I mostly mixed it with finely diced cartilage but has occasionally used finely diced fat, especially in revision cases. In contrast, patients with thick skin should undergo a further assessment of their skin to determine which dermatological treatments are more suitable for enhancing their final results. This may include skin care regimens, topical retinoic acid,

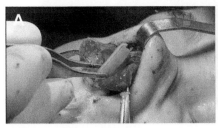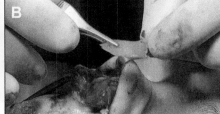

Fig. 2. (*A–B*) Septal extension graft.

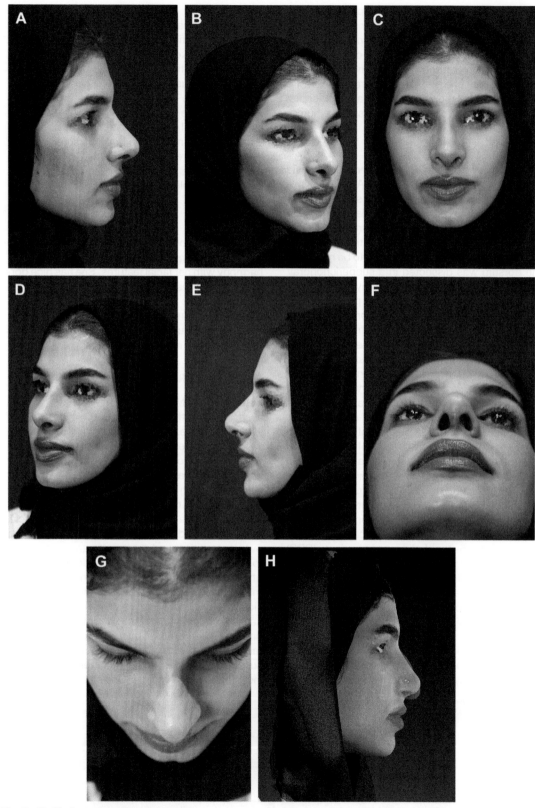

Fig. 3. (*A–H*): Postoperative patient views.

oral isotretinoin, radiofrequency, and resurfacing procedures.[11,12] It also alters the choice of surgical techniques used as a more structural approach is preferred with more use of grafts to push against the skin envelope, hence enhancing the definition. Along with direct skin thinning, defatting, or excision of SMAS layer (superficial musculoaponeurotic system) in some cases.

With the reemerging popularity of preservation rhinoplasty techniques, a lot of Middle Eastern patients are potential candidates with the combination of strong cartilages and medium skin thickness. In patients with thicker skin, tip preservation techniques may not yield satisfactory results as a more structural approach is preferred. However, dorsal preservation techniques can be helpful with a lot of these patients, giving a more "natural" dorsum which is preferred by most patients. In this case, we elected not to preserve the nasal dorsum as the patient had a prominent supra tip depression, along with a wide nasal dorsum and a small cartilaginous hump, so a more "classic" way of hump resection was used.

CLINICS CARE POINTS

- In dealing with the Middle Eastern population, the rhinoplasty surgeon should be aware of the history, ideologies, and demographics of the Middle East.
- Ideal nasal shape varies greatly between different Middle Eastern regions, the surgeon should clarify with each patient his/her expected outcome of surgery.
- Although many patients ask for a more Caucasian-like nose, most of them still want a nose that fits their racial background, that is, a modest increase in rotation and conservative dorsal reduction are common requests, especially among male patients.
- In most of the Middle Eastern territories, a straight rather than a scooped dorsum is ideal for male patients, although younger female individuals are becoming more in favor of a slightly lower dorsum.
- Although the bony facial structure, nasal and septal cartilages tend to be quite similar, the skin quality and thickness vary widely among different groups in the Middle East.
- A lot of emphasis in the Gulf region is put on how narrow the nose is, narrow tip and thin dorsum with a narrow alar base are considered ideal "straight like a sword." In contrast, cephalically oriented lower lateral cartilages, slight under rotation and a small hump are well tolerated.

- Be aware of thick, sebaceous, rhinophyma-like skin which is not uncommon, especially in northern Africa.
- The surgeon should have extensive knowledge of dermatological treatment options to enhance the skin soft tissue envelope.
- The rhinoplasty surgeon should be aware of different rhinoplasty approaches and techniques. This is especially important for young surgeons starting their career if they deal frequently Middle Eastern patients.

SUPPLEMENTARY DATA

Supplementary data related to this article can be found online at https://doi.org/10.1016/j.fsc.2022.07.006.

REFERENCES

1. Available at: https://en.wikipedia.org/wiki/List_of_Middle_Eastern_countries_by_population. Accessed January 2022.
2. Azizzadeh B, Mashkevich G. Middle eastern rhinoplasty. Facial Plast Surg Clin 2010;18(1):201–6.
3. Apaydin F. Rhinoplasty in the middle eastern nose. Facial Plast Surg Clin North Am 2014;22(3):349–55.
4. Rohrich RJ, Ghavami A. Rhinoplasty for middle eastern noses. Plast Reconstr Surg 2009;123(4):1343–54.
5. Al-Qattan MM, Alsaeed AA, Al-Madani OK, et al. Anthropometry of the saudi arabian nose. J Craniofac Surg 2012;23(3):821–4.
6. Ozdemir F, Uzun A. Anthropometric analysis of the nose in young Turkish men and women. J Cranio-Maxillofacial Surg 2015;43(7):1244–7.
7. Heidari Z, Mahmoudzadeh-Sagheb H, Khammar T, et al. Anthropometric measurements of the external nose in 18–25-year-old Sistani and Baluch aborigine women in the southeast of Iran. Folia morphologica 2009;68(2):88–92.
8. Daniel RK. Rhinoplasty: a simplified, three-stitch, open tip suture technique. Part I: primary rhinoplasty. Plast Reconstr Surg 1999;103(5):1491–502.
9. Davis RE. Lateral crural tensioning for refinement of the wide and underprojected nasal tip: rethinking the lateral crural steal. Facial Plast Surg Clin 2015;23(1):23–53.
10. Kovacevic M, Riedel F, Wurm J, et al. Cartilage scales embedded in fibrin gel. Facial Plast Surg 2017;33(02):225–32.
11. Kosins AM, Obagi ZE. Managing the difficult soft tissue envelope in facial and rhinoplasty surgery. Aesthet Surg J 2017;37(2):143–57.
12. Cobo R, Camacho JG, Orrego J. Integrated management of the thick-skinned rhinoplasty patient. Facial Plast Surg 2018;34(01):003–8.

Rhinoplasty Considerations in the Ethnic Patient
The East-Asian Patients

Marn Joon Park, MD, Yong Ju Jang, MD, PhD*

KEYWORDS

- East asian rhinoplasty • Deviated nasal septum • Hump nose • Short nose • Revision rhinoplasty
- Dorsal convexity • Dorsal augmentation

KEY POINTS

- Augmentation is one of the most important considerations in the rhinoplasty of East Asian patients.
- Building a strong supporting structure in the septal framework is the key element for successful augmentation.
- With the frequent usage of silicone implants in East Asian rhinoplasty, the surgeon should properly address the possible long-term adverse outcomes of silicone implants. Nasal deviation due to the displacement of the silicone implant or deformed and shortened nose due to the contracture in the tissues surrounding the silicone implant are the 2 most important features.

INTRODUCTION

The crucial importance of augmentation rhinoplasty should be considered when consultation for or undertaking rhinoplasty in the Asian population. The relatively flat East Asian nasal profile indicates the key role of the augmentation rhinoplasty process in achieving a satisfactory cosmetic outcome, and in addition to augmentation, correction of the deviation, hump, saddle, and short nose deformity should be adequately performed.[1]

Understanding the anatomic differences between the East Asian nose and the Caucasian nose is a key prerequisite for corrective surgery because the nasal anatomy of the East Asian patient differs from that of the Caucasian patient.[2] The East Asian patient tends to have thicker skin with more pronounced subcutaneous soft tissue as well as low nasal tip height and weak support from the lower lateral cartilages (LLCs). Moreover, the height of the dorsum and radix is often very low, and this is accompanied by a smaller, shorter, and thicker nasal bone.[3] Furthermore, the septal cartilage is often very thin and small, which leaves an inadequate amount of cartilage for use as graft materials for providing structural support or dorsal augmentation, and necessitates the harvesting of additional cartilage for grafting. A unique challenge of rhinoplasty in the East Asian patients is that the surgeon must be capable of appropriately managing silicone-implant-related complications as displacement, infection, and secondary deformity due to contracture are major complications of silicone rhinoplasty.

In this article, we describe the surgical procedure and outcome in 4 representative cases: augmentation of a flat nose, hump and deviated nose, revision rhinoplasty in a patient with deviated nose, and severely contracted nose.

Department of Otorhinolaryngology-Head and Neck Surgery, Asan Medical Center, University of Ulsan College of Medicine, 388-1 Pungnap 2-dong, Songpa-gu, Seoul 138-736, Republic of Korea
* Corresponding author.
E-mail address: 3712yjjang@gmail.com

Facial Plast Surg Clin N Am 30 (2022) 527–540
https://doi.org/10.1016/j.fsc.2022.07.007
1064-7406/22/© 2022 Elsevier Inc. All rights reserved.

facialplastic.theclinics.com

CASE STUDY/PRESENTATION
Case 1. Primary Rhinoplasty for the Correction of Flat Nose

Case presentation
A 36-year-old woman visited the clinic with complaints of a flat nose and symptomatic nasal septal deviation. The patient had poorly developed nasal bone as well as weak support from the upper lateral cartilage (ULC) and septum, which caused shortening, flattening, and concavity of the nasal dorsum (**Fig. 1**A). The patient had relatively thick skin and underdeveloped alar cartilages, which manifested as a poorly defined, underprojected tip. Moreover, slightly retracted columella and an increased nasolabial angle were noticeable. During the preoperative consultation, the patient expressed a desire for a more elongated nose with an adequately projected tip and well-augmented dorsum, ultimately creating a balanced brow-tip-dorsal esthetic line. For the tip, the patient demanded mild derotation and better definition and projection.

Operative procedures
Under general anesthesia, the skin–soft tissue envelope was elevated through an inverted V-shaped transcolumellar and marginal incision (**Fig. 2**). Elevation of the bilateral septal mucoperichondrial flap revealed thin, weakened, and poorly developed septal cartilage deviated to the right side. After ensuring the preservation of sufficient septal cartilage for an L-strut, the deviated septal cartilage, vomer, and perpendicular plate of the ethmoid (PPE) was resected and harvested. For augmentation, the patient's sixth costal cartilage was harvested and designed into strip-like pieces that were used as bilateral extended spreader grafts (ESGs) on both sides of the dorsal septum. A caudal septal extension graft (CSEG) was sandwiched between the ESGs in an end-to-end relationship with the caudal septum, simultaneously derotating and projecting the tip. The ULCs were reapproximated to the septum–ESG complex using 4 to 0 polydioxanone suture (PDS), and the LLCs were sutured to the CSEG to project and slightly derotate the tip. We found that the tip needed more augmentation to meet the desired esthetic goal, and therefore, 2 layers of tip graft were added for additional tip projection and tip definition. After elevating the nasal tip, dorsal augmentation was undertaken using a

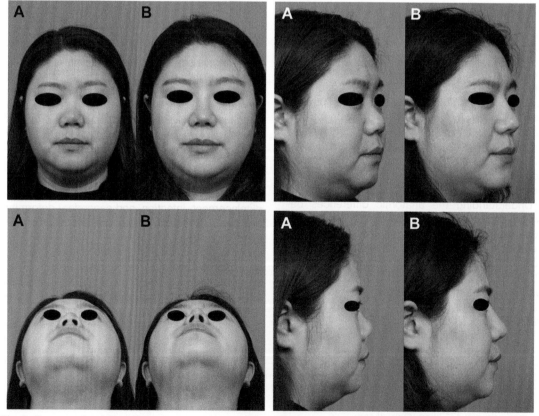

Fig. 1. Preoperative (*A*) and 1 year postoperative (*B*) photographs of a patient with flat nose. The short, flat dorsum with underprojected, poor tip definition was successfully augmented, as seen in the postoperative image.

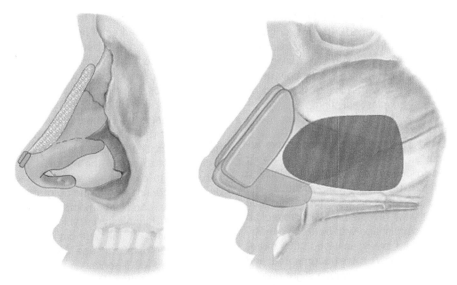

Fig. 2. The surgical procedures for case No. 1. Bilateral extended spreader grafts, caudal septal extension graft, glued-and-diced costal cartilage dorsal implant, and multilayered tip graft were inserted for dorsal augmentation and tip projection.

glued-diced costal cartilage implant that was shaped with a Jang cartilage mold as follows (**Fig. 3**): to create the dorsal implant, cadaveric fascia lata (California Transplant Services, Inc., Carlsbad, CA, USA) measuring approximately 4 × 1 cm was obtained and designed to provide the dorsal surface of the implant. Fibrin glue (Greenplast Q, GC Pharma Co., Ltd., Republic of Korea) was then applied between 2 and 3 layers of diced costal cartilage. The cap of the mold was assembled, and the mold was manually compressed to drain out excess fluid and glue. Using a

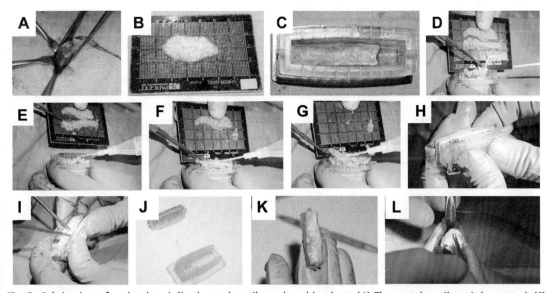

Fig. 3. Fabrication of a glued-and-diced costal cartilage dorsal implant. (*A*) The costal cartilage is harvested. (*B*) Harvested costal cartilage is diced. (*C*) The perichondrium was separated from the costal cartilage, and layered on the bottom of the 3D-printed cartilage mold. (*D–G*) Afterward, the mold is filled with layers of diced costal cartilage with fibrin glue. (*H, I*) The cap of the mold is closed, and the mold is compressed to drain out the excessive fluid within the implant. (*J, K*) The implant is taken out of the mold. (*L*) The fabricated implant is being inserted in the dorsum. On insertion, the surface of perichondrium or fascia should face the dorsal aspect, to achieve a natural looking dorsal line.

4 cm × 3 mm-mold, a dorsal implant of the corresponding size was fashioned. The implant was carefully inserted over the nasal dorsum, following full exposure of the nasal dorsum using the retractor and skin hooks. The transcolumellar and marginal incisions were closed, followed by nasal taping and Aquaplast splinting.

Postoperative outcome

The patient had an uneventful postoperative recovery without any complications. At the 1-year postoperative follow-up, an esthetically pleasing and well-defined brow-tip-dorsal esthetic line with improved tip definition was noticeable (see **Fig. 1**B). Basal view revealed that improved tip projection and nostril shape with better symmetry and orientation had been achieved. On three-quarter and lateral view, a well-augmented and straight dorsal line was noted with a slight degree of derotation. Additionally, a subtle supratip break in the dorsal line aided a more natural-looking feminine appearance in this patient.

Discussion

There is vast diversity in the shape of the East Asian nose. Case 1 typifies a fraction of patients who require significant dorsum and tip augmentation. Augmentation of the nose should commence with the lower-third of the tip, and septal extension grafts constitute a reliable and robust option for augmenting this region. Among the various techniques of septal extension grafting, we prefer expanding the L-strut and the caudal septal framework through a combination of bilateral ESGs with unilateral CSEGs in an end-to-end fashion (**Fig. 4**). In most cases, the septal cartilage is relatively weak and is present in inadequate quantities to properly augment the septal cartilage framework.[4–6] Therefore, when selecting the grafting material, we prefer to use the costal cartilage due to its abundance and strength. Septal extension grafts are hidden grafts that can avoid the

common complication of tip graft showing. However, when the degree of projection is inadequate and the patient needs better definition of the tip due to thicker skin, additional tip grafting is needed. Tip grafting techniques that are useful in Asians include the shied graft, multilayer tip grafts, and tip onlay grafting (**Fig. 5**). The grafting method should be selected from the characteristics of the native anatomy of the tip cartilage and the esthetic goal of the patients. When placing the tip grafts, it is important to soften the margin by meticulous carving or to camouflage with crushed cartilage or perichondrium around the tip grafts.

Adequate dorsal augmentation highlights the essence of rhinoplasty in typical East-Asian patients. Based on the authors' experience, the glued-diced costal cartilage dorsal implant using a mold (see **Fig. 3**) serves as a reliable option for dorsal augmentation. Dorsal augmentation using the diced cartilage has increasingly gained popularity these days because it can provide a natural, esthetically pleasing dorsal line and sufficiently augment the dorsum.[7–11] As shown in the photograph obtained at the 1-year postoperative follow-up of this patient, the described method allows the creation of a natural-looking dorsal line, with minimal risk for dorsal implant migration or warping.[12]

CASE 2. CORRECTION OF HUMP AND DEVIATED NOSE
Case Presentation

A 21-year-old man visited the clinic with a complaint of a hump and deviated nose. The patient had a history of nasal trauma that was previously managed with a closed reduction in another clinic 8 years ago. On examination, the patient had a nasal septum that deviated to the left side as well as corresponding nasal obstruction. In the frontal view, there was a left-sided nasal bony axis deviation and a right-sided cartilaginous deviation (**Fig. 6**A). Basal view revealed the relatively low

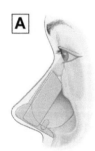
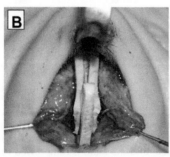
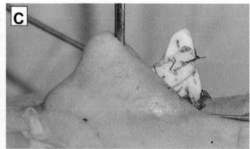

Fig. 4. (*A*) Caudal septal extension graft (CSE), which was sandwiched between the bilateral extended spreader grafts. The CSE was placed in an end-to-end relationship with the caudal septum. Intraoperative image of the frontal (*B*) and lateral aspect (*C*).

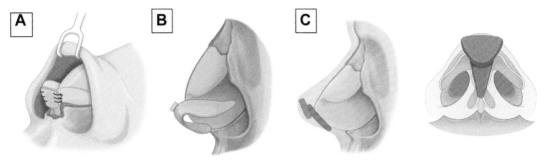

Fig. 5. Various tip graft techniques for improving tip esthetics. (*A*) Shield graft. (*B*) Tip onlay graft. (*C*) Multilayer tip grafts. First, a shield graft is placed, projecting the tip. Second, another graft is added on top of the shield graft.

tip height. On the three-quarter and lateral view, dorsal convexity was noticeable around the rhinion area.

Operative Procedures

Under general anesthesia, open rhinoplasty was undertaken through an inverted V-shaped trans-columellar and marginal incision. Ensuring septal L-strut structure preservation, the deviated septal cartilage, vomer, and PPE were resected and harvested (**Fig. 7**). The bony hump was reduced with manual rasping of the nasal bone and uncapping of the underlying cartilaginous hump (**Fig. 8**). Next, the cartilaginous hump in line with the dorsal septum was resected incrementally, and the overriding ULCS are gently trimmed out. A bony batten graft, which was created using the

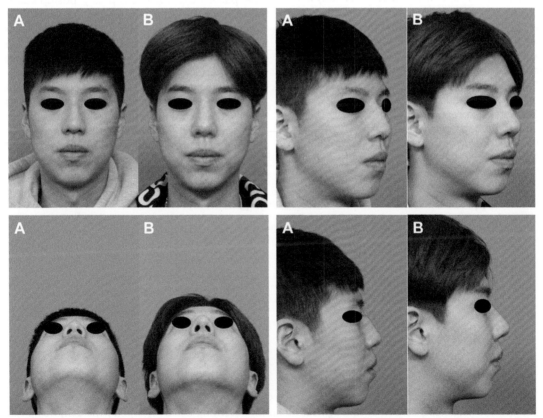

Fig. 6. (*A*) Preoperative and 1-year postoperative (*B*) photographs of a patient with deviated and hump nose. The convexity in the dorsal line is straightened with adequately augmented dorsum and projected tip, as seen in the 1-year postoperative photograph.

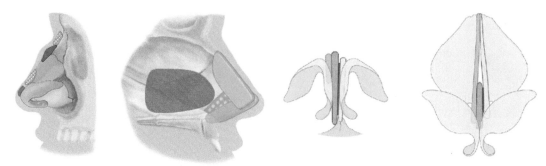

Fig. 7. Rhinoplasty on deviated and hump nose patient. (Case No.2). The hump reduction was done with cartilaginous hump removal followed by rasping of the bony cap. Bony batten graft was inserted on the right caudal septum. An extended spreader graft and a caudal septal extension graft was inserted on the right side of the native septal cartilage, centering the left-side deviated nose more to the right side. A tip onlay graft was inserted.

harvested septal bone, was placed on the right side of the caudal septum to straighten and strengthen the deviated caudal septum. In this patient, the amount, thickness, and strength of the septal cartilage were sufficient enough to be designed as the structural graft materials. Therefore, using the harvested septal cartilage, one CSEG was placed in a side-to-side relationship with the caudal septum, lateral to the already fixed bony batten graft. Then, an ESG was inserted at the right side of the dorsal septum, and the caudal end was placed at the lateral side of the CSE. Using this grafting technique, the cartilaginous axis deviation directed to the left side was corrected (**Fig. 9**). The ULCs were reapproximated to the dorsal septum, and the LLCs centered by the CSE were also reapproximated. We ascertained that a slight degree of tip projection was needed; therefore, one piece of the leftover septal cartilage was designed into a tip onlay graft and sutured to

the domal area of the tip (**Fig. 10**). Finally, to soften the dorsal line, segmental dorsal augmentation with camouflage graft using the crushed leftover septal cartilages was placed over the radix and supratip.

Postoperative Outcome

The patient did not develop any postoperative complications. At the 1-year postoperative follow-up, we observed that a wider nasal dorsum with a more defined brow-tip-dorsal esthetic line was achieved and resulted in an esthetically more masculine facial appearance (see **Fig. 6**B). The tip height had increased, the columella had straightened, and symmetric nostril size was achieved. On the three-quarter and the lateral view, the dorsal convexity had disappeared and a new straight dorsal line with increased tip height had been achieved.

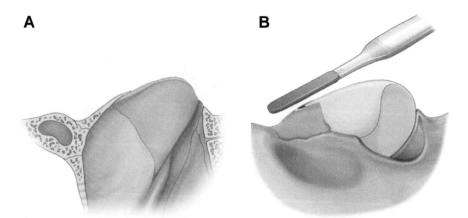

Fig. 8. (A) The nasal hump consists of cartilaginous hump with overlying thin bony cap. (B) The bony hump was reduced with manual rasping of the nasal bone and uncapping of the underlying cartilaginous hump. Next, the cartilaginous hump in line with the dorsal septum was resected incrementally, and the overriding ULCS are gently trimmed out.

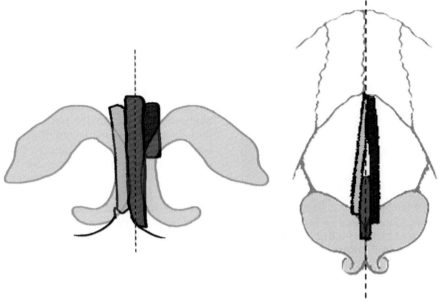

Fig. 9. Deviated nose correction of the low thirds can be achieved by redirecting the center of the nose. The right-sided cartilaginous deviation (in green) is corrected by placing the extended spreader graft (in blue) with caudal septal extension graft (in red) on the opposite side of the deviation.

Discussion

In this case, correction of dorsal convexity and the deviated nose was successfully achieved. Although not as prevalent as in rhinoplasty of Caucasian patients, the correction of a hump nose poses a significant problem in the rhinoplasty of East Asian patients. East Asians generally prefer a nose with a prominent tip and well-augmented nasal dorsum, and the concept of redistribution is important. Hump reduction should be undertaken conservatively and incrementally, including careful removal of the bony cap and the cartilaginous hump. Tip augmentation using a septal

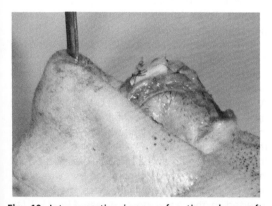

Fig. 10. Intraoperative image of a tip onlay graft. Following hump reduction, tip onlay grafting is a recommended procedure to prevent concavity in the dorsal line in hump nose rhinoplasty.

extension graft is an essential maneuver to achieve an esthetically pleasing tip height. Midvault reconstruction with a spreader graft or a spreader flap and camouflage grafts are essential maneuvers to successfully ensure esthetic outcomes. Following hump reduction, the next step is to focus on addressing the septal deviation and reinforcing septal structural strength.[13] The deviation of the caudal septum in this patient was successfully managed with a bony batten graft created from the harvested septal bones that was placed contralateral to the caudal septal deviation (**Fig. 11**). Based on our clinical experience, the authors have found that the described method above is an effective method for correcting caudal septal deviation. Patients with a hump nose frequently have a combined deformity of a deviated nose, for which placement of the caudal septal extension grafting in a side-to-side manner (batten type) may be appropriate.[14–19] A unilateral batten-type CSEG is placed on the side contralateral to the septal deviation, then situated diagonally across the caudal septum toward the nasal tip, and sutured to the septum. Subsequently, a unilateral ESG is sutured contralateral to the septal deviation with its caudal border and the native dorsal septum sandwiching the CSEG. Splaying of the ESG adds additional volume to the concave nasal sidewall and makes the nose seem straighter (see **Fig. 9**). This patient had a relatively large and strong septal cartilage, which enabled the creation of adequate grafts for the reconstruction of the

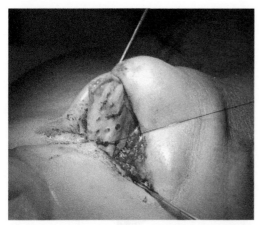

Fig. 11. The bony batten placed on the opposite side of the caudal septal deviation aided in straightening the caudal septum and structural support in the caudal septum.

septal framework. However, in cases of thinned, damaged, or undeveloped septal cartilage, the surgeon should consider using autologous costal cartilage for various grafting.

To create an esthetically pleasing dorsal line, the balance between the height of the reduced nasal bone and the tip should be achieved. Additional tip grafting is required when tip projection using a CSEG cannot achieve the desired height in moderate-to-thick-skinned individuals. The majority of convex noses seem long; therefore, it its crucial not to create a longer-looking nose because of a tip graft in hump nose patients. Shield grafts are an excellent tip-projection method but tend to increase the length of the nose by providing additional volume on the nasal lobule. Therefore, tip onlay grafting on the nasal dome is a preferred method because it provides additional tip projection with a slightly rotated appearance of the tip, which is more favorable for patients with dorsal convexity (see **Fig. 10**).

CASE 3. REVISION RHINOPLASTY IN THE DEVIATED NOSE DUE TO DISPLACED SILICONE DORSAL IMPLANT
Case Presentation

A 27-year-old woman visited the clinic with a complaint of deviated nose. The patient had undergone rhinoplasty, using a septal cartilage graft and prefabricated silicone implant, at another clinic 13 years before the visit to our clinic. The patient reported that her nose gradually seemed deviated after the rhinoplasty, and she developed symptoms of nasal obstruction especially on the right side, following orthognatic 2-jaw surgery. The patient was relatively satisfied with the current

dorsal height and tip height but wanted to correct the deviated appearance of the nose.

Nasal endoscopy revealed caudal septal deviation to the right. In the preoperative frontal photograph (**Fig. 12**), the axis of the nose is deviated to the right side, with a slight retraction of the columella, which results in decreased nostril show. On basal view, the tip height was relatively low, along with an asymmetric nostril. On lateral and three-quarter view, the height of the dorsum was relatively balanced with regard to the tip, and a straight dorsal line was observed. Notably, the axial image in the patient's preoperative facial computed tomographic scan revealed that the dorsal silicone implant had displaced more to the left of the nasal dorsum (**Fig. 13**).

Operative procedures

Under general anesthesia, the skin–soft tissue envelope was elevated through an inverted V-shaped transcolumellar and marginal incision (**Fig. 14**). During flap elevation, a prefabricated silicone implant over the nasal dorsum was identified and removed), which revealed a defect in the bony dorsum. Bilateral medial and lateral osteotomy and subsequent medialization of the triangular bony segment on both sides were undertaken to correct the deviated bony axis and to close the open roof caused by the previous surgery. On elevation of the septal mucoperichondrial flap, a columellar strut graft, which was inserted during the previous rhinoplasty, was seen and removed; the caudal septal deviation was noticeable in the nasal septum. Using the cutting and suture technique, the most angulated portion of the caudal septal cartilage was cut and sutured again after slightly overlapping the upper and lower segments (**Fig. 15**). A cartilaginous batten graft was placed on the left side of the caudal septum for further support. To straighten and augment the cartilaginous septum, the patient's sixth costal cartilage was harvested. Bilateral ESGs were placed on both sides of the dorsal septal cartilage, and caudal septal cartilage extension graft was positioned between 2 ESGs, in an end-to-end manner. After closuring the ULC and LLC using sutures, a tip graft made of diced costal cartilage wrapped in harvested costal perichondrium was placed at the tip. Similarly as in Case 1, using a cartilage mold (4 cm length and 2 mm thickness), a dorsal implant with diced costal cartilage that was glued and capped with fascia lata was created and inserted in the nasal dorsum (see **Fig. 5**). With the remaining diced costal cartilage, a camouflage graft was inserted over the right supratip for the correction of the subtle remaining deviation.

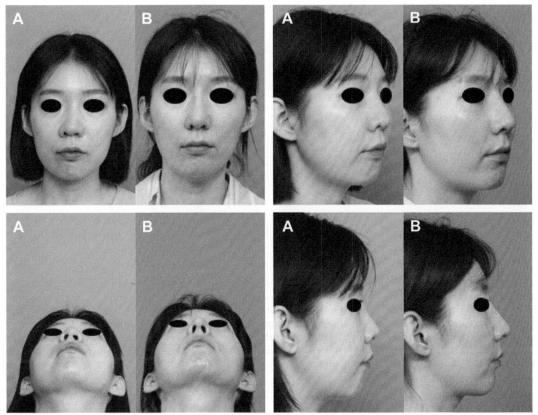

Fig. 12. **(A)** Preoperative and one year postoperative **(B)** photographs of a patient with a previous history of silicone rhinoplasty. The dorsal center is slightly shifted to the left side, and cartilaginous dorsum is deviated to the right side. The patient underwent revision rhinoplasty for the deviated nose. A 1-year postoperative photo reveals successful correction of the nasal deviation. The dorsal silicone implant removed, and replaced with glued-diced costal cartilage dorsal implant.

Postoperative Outcome

The postoperative course was uneventful. At the 1-year postoperative follow-up visit, correction of the deviated nose with an esthetically pleasing brow-tip-dorsal line was successfully achieved (see **Fig. 12**B). On basal view, the tip projection resulted in esthetically satisfying tip definition and symmetry in the nostril size and shape. The

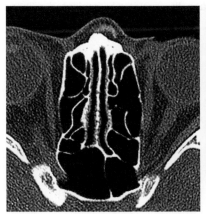
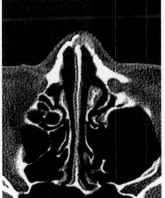
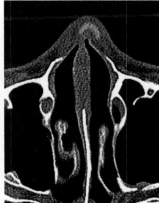

Fig. 13. In an axial cut in the computed tomograph image, dorsal silicone implant positioned more to the left side on the dorsum is noticeable.

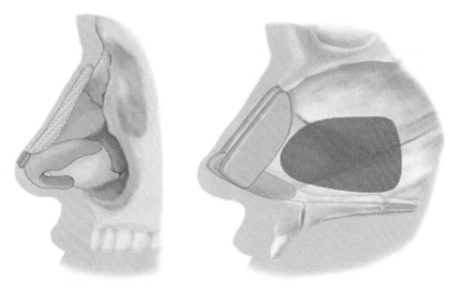

Fig. 14. The surgical procedures performed in revision rhinoplasty for the deviated nose (case No. 3). Following the removal of the dorsal silicone implant, the deviation of the nasal bone with open roof deformity caused by previous rhinoplasty was noticed. Bilateral medial and lateral osteotomy were made to medialize the bony pyramid and to correct the bony axis. Caudal septal cartilage extension graft was positioned between 2 extended spreader grafts in an end-to-end manner. Diced costal cartilage wrapped with costal perichondrium was placed at the tip, and tip camouflage graft with crushed cartilage was inserted on supratip. Glued diced costal cartilage dorsal implant was inserted for the dorsal augmentation.

three-quarter and lateral view showed a straight dorsal line with minimal augmentation in dorsal height compared with the appearance evident in the preoperative photograph, and the outcome matched the patient's preoperative cosmetic requirement. The slight elongation in the columella helped in increasing the nostril show as well as decreasing the nasolabial angle, resulting in a cosmetically desirable outcome.

Discussion

One of the common issues with a dorsal implant, such as a silicone implant, is its unpredictability.

There is a possibility that dorsal implants may migrate in the dorsal pocket during wound healing, which creates an unexpected shifting, resulting in nasal deviation in the long-term postoperative period.[20–24] In cases of revision rhinoplasty in which a silicone implant was previously inserted, it is important to address the nasal deformity after complete removal of the silicone implant. After properly managing the nasal deformity, dorsal augmentation with the previously inserted silicone implant or other autologous tissue implants (ie, diced costal cartilage) can be simultaneously achieved if there are no signs of infection. We prefer to replace the previously implanted silicone

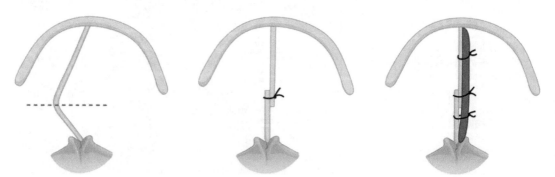

Fig. 15. Placement of the bypass L-strut graft (integrated costal cartilage columella-dorsal implant) using the autologous costal cartilage.

implant with autologous tissue. In cases with evident infection around the dorsal implant, a staged operation is required because a single-stage operation confers a higher risk of postoperative infection, with disastrous outcomes. In this case, we did not notice any signs of infection around the previously inserted silicone implant and accordingly performed single-stage rhinoplasty. The removal of the silicone implant revealed an open-roof deformity in the nasal bony cap, with a right-sided deviation in the bony and cartilaginous axis, that may have been caused by the previous surgical hump removal or due to resorption of the nasal bone due to the longstanding pressure exerted by the silicone implant on the underlying nasal bone. Therefore, appropriate osteotomies and manual narrowing of the nasal bone were used to correct the open-roof deformity. Many patients present with a deviated nose with a silicone graft in their nasal dorsum; the deviation is usually due to the displacement of the silicone implant or because of an underlying nasal skeletal deviation. In this case, even after the removal of the silicone implant, the nose looked deviated, which necessitated specific maneuvers to correct the deviated nose. Correction of cartilaginous deviation is a challenging task wherein several different maneuvers are needed for perfecting the surgical outcome. Correction of the cartilaginous deviation should begin by straightening and strengthening the deviated caudal septum. In this case, the caudal septal deviation was corrected by adopting the cutting and suture technique that was originally developed by the corresponding author (see **Fig. 15**). The rationale for this technique is that the excess length of the caudal septal cartilage is the main abnormality in this type of deviation. Thus, cutting and overlapping of the most convex part of the caudal septal L-strut could reduce the excess length, thereby creating a straight caudal septal segment but without affecting the original tip height. The placement of bilateral spreader grafts is the most popular and reliable method of straightening the dorsal L-strut (see **Fig. 4**). In this case, we placed bilateral spreader grafts with thick costal cartilage, which ensured sound support of the lower two-thirds of the nose. In this case, tip augmentation was achieved by a CSEG and additional grafting with perichondrium-wrapped diced cartilage. Fascia or perichondrium-wrapped diced cartilage constitutes a good option for tip augmentation that decreases the risk of tip graft showing and confers better capability of creating a natural-looking tip shape that softly blends with the thinner tip skin.

CASE 4. REVISION RHINOPLASTY IN THE SHORTENED, DEFORMED NOSE WITH A PREVIOUS SILICONE RHINOPLASTY
Case Presentation

A 29-year-old man visited the clinic with an upturned nasal deformity and a history of having undergone 2 rhinoplasties. The patient underwent a primary rhinoplasty, using autologous ear cartilage, in another clinic 10 years ago and subsequently underwent revision rhinoplasty with a silicone implant 7 years ago in another clinic. A few months before the initial visit, due to repeated inflammation, the patient underwent removal of the silicone implant in the other clinic.

On frontal view, an upturned and shortened nose with increased nostril show was noticeable along with pinched and asymmetric nostrils (**Fig. 16**A). The brow-tip-dorsal esthetic line was very wide and indistinct. On basal view, the columella was tilted to the right side, and the discrepancy in the size and shape of bilateral nostrils were noticeable. On three-quarter and lateral view, a severely upturned nasal tip with a wide nasolabial angle was seen, and the radix and dorsal height were very low, which resulted in the severe concavity of the nasal dorsum. There was a polly beak-like prominence on the supratip cartilaginous dorsum. During the preoperative consultation, the patient expressed a very high esthetic goal, which he desired to have a completely normal looking new nose, without any stigmata of the contracted nose.

Operative Procedure

Under general anesthesia, the skin–soft tissue envelope was elevated via an inverted V-shaped transcolumellar and marginal incision (**Fig. 17**). The elevation of the skin flap was extremely difficult due to severe scarring. On flap elevation, the nasal bone showed an open-roof deformity, which was especially prominent on the left side. The absence of the quadrangular cartilage was suspected on palpation, and the severe adhesion in the septal mucosa hindered the complete mucoperichondrial flap dissection of the nasal septum; therefore, partial dissection of the right dorsal septum was performed. Because the patient had a high septal deviation due to a PPE deviation, an endonasal septal incision immediately before the deviated portion was made under endoscopic guidance, and the deviated septal bone was resected and the partially raised flap was redraped. The harvested septal bone was designed for the bony batten graft and placed to the right of the caudal septum. The sixth costal cartilage was harvested through a 2-cm incision.

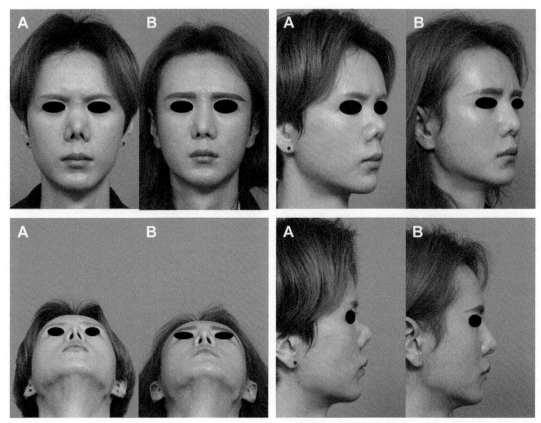

Fig. 16. (A) Preoperative and one year postoperative (B) photographs of a patient with in a patient with previous history of multiple rhinoplasty using the prefabricated silicone dorsal implant. The severely deformed, shortened, and up-turned nose is noticeable. A 1-year postoperative photo reveals successful reconstruction of the nasal deformity in this patient. In the frontal view, the starting point of the nose had moved much higher, and the excessive nostril show seen in the preoperative photograph was considerably decreased. In the basal view, the tilted columella was corrected and the tip height had increased. The shape and size of the nostril was markedly symmetric. On three-quarter and lateral view, a well-balanced profile line is achieved as a result of dorsal augmentation, tip derotation, and elongation of the retracted columella.

Preoperatively, we planned to derotate the lower third by releasing the fibrotic tissue between the upper lateral and LLC followed by strong reinforcement with ESG and CSEG complex to anchor the released alar cartilages. However, in this case, excessive scarring of the septal mucosa and an inability to create a complete septal mucoperichondrial pocket, which hampered the placement of the bilateral ESGs and CSEG. Thus, instead of reinforcing and elongating the native septum with bilateral ESG and CSE, a bypass L-strut graft made of the costal cartilage (integrated costal cartilage columella-dorsal implant) was designed to provide strong structural support to the lower two-thirds of the nose, whereby the released LLCs were anchored (**Fig. 18**).[25] The defect in the nasal bone was reconstructed with the perichondrium of the harvested costal cartilage as well as multiple layers of additional homologous

fascia. A shield graft was placed on the tip, and dorsal augmentation was achieved using glued-and-diced costal cartilage dorsal implant created by using the same mold as described earlier, followed by covering with the costal cartilage perichondrium. Finally, remnant diced costal cartilage was inserted into the radix, supratip, and tip for camouflage grafting.

Postoperative Outcome

The patient recovered without any postoperative complications. At the 1-year postoperative follow-up visit, we observed that the shortened and upturned nasal deformity was successfully corrected and a more defined and esthetically pleasing brow-tip-dorsal line was achieved (**Fig. 12**B). In the frontal view, the starting point of the nose had moved much higher, and the

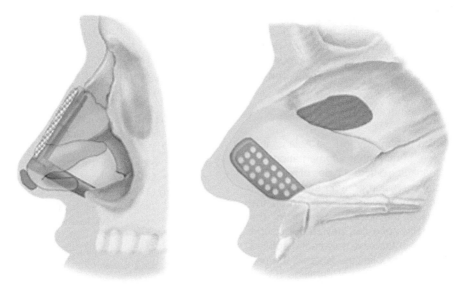

Fig. 17. The surgical procedures performed in case No. 4. A bony batten graft was inserted using the harvested bone of the PPE. A bypass L-strut graft (Integrated costal cartilage columella-dorsal implant) made with costal cartilage was inserted, followed by shield graft insertion on the tip. Dorsal augmentation with remaining diced costal cartilage grafting was done on the radix, supratip, and tip.

excessive nostril show seen in the preoperative photograph was considerably decreased. In the basal view, the tilted columella was corrected and the tip height had increased. The shape and size of the nostril was markedly symmetric. On three-quarter and lateral view, we noted that dorsal augmentation, derotation of the nasal tip, and elongation of the retracted columella were achieved to form a well-balanced profile line.

Discussion

This patient presented with a severe upturning and shortening of the nose due to multiple previous rhinoplasties using silicone implants, and this deformity was nicely corrected with a bypass-L graft using the autologous costal cartilage. A short nose is one of the most difficult deformities to correct, and the aim of corrective surgery is the actual

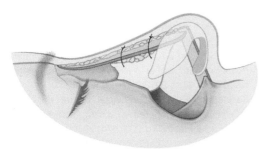

Fig. 18. Placement of the bypass L-strut graft (integrated costal cartilage columella-dorsal implant) using the autologous costal cartilage.

extension of the nasal length with the simultaneous creation of an illusion of a longer-looking nose. Short noses should be corrected by adhering to the surgical principles of lengthening the central and lateral segments, tip grafting to lengthen the nose, and dorsal augmentation. In most cases, to elongate the central compartment, the authors prefer placing the end-to-end type CSEG sandwiched between bilateral ESGs (see **Fig. 4**). However, in cases which dissection of the septal mucoperichondrium is impossible due to severe scarring, any attempt to dissect the septal mucosa carries an increased risk of further injury to the already damaged septal mucosa, as in this case. In this difficult scenario, using an integrated dorsal implant and columellar strut allows surgeons to bypass the problematic cartilaginous septum and enables reconstruction in the lower two-thirds of the nose. To create an integrated dorsal implant and columellar strut from costal cartilage, one monoblock dorsal implant is sutured to a columellar strut to form the new cartilaginous L strut (see **Fig. 18**A). The dorsal implant part can be inserted directly into the subperiosteal pocket above the nasal bone and spans the nasal dorsum. The columellar strut should be sutured in front of the anterior nasal spine or simply be inserted into the space between the divided medial crura (see **Fig. 18**B). If lengthening of the central compartment is not combined with adequate lengthening of the lateral compartment, the nose may look pinched and unnatural. It is therefore important to address the lateral compartment of the nose accordingly to attain an esthetically harmonious surgical outcome. As a short nose is usually accompanied by a concave nasal dorsum, dorsal augmentation is a crucial surgical procedure because the nose seems longer after the correction of the dorsal concavity.

SUMMARY

When performing rhinoplasty in East Asians, it is important to bear in mind that augmentation is a key factor for managing different types of nasal deformities. Septal extension grafting and spreader grafts are crucial maneuvers for building up the lower two-thirds of the nose, especially for the successful correction of a flat, deviated, or short nose. Dorsal augmentation is universally applied in almost all Asian rhinoplasties, wherein the use of glue-diced autologous costal cartilage dorsal implant has played an increasingly important role. For successful correction of the Asian hump nose, conservative hump reduction coupled with appropriate midvault reconstruction, radix augmentation, and tip augmentation should be performed.

DISCLOSURE

The authors have nothing to disclose.

ACKNOWLEDGMENTS

None.

REFERENCES

1. Jang YJ, Yi JS. Perspectives in asian rhinoplasty. Facial Plast Surg 2014;30(2):123–30.
2. Jang YJ, Yu MS. Rhinoplasty for the Asian nose. Facial Plast Surg 2010;26(2):93–101.
3. Wang JH, Jang YJ, Park SK, et al. Measurement of aesthetic proportions in the profile view of Koreans. Ann Plast Surg 2009;62(2):109–13.
4. Kim JS, Khan NA, Song HM, et al. Intraoperative measurements of harvestable septal cartilage in rhinoplasty. Ann Plast Surg 2010;65(6):519–23.
5. Jang YJ, Kim SH. Tip Grafting for the Asian Nose. Facial Plast Surg Clin North Am 2018;26(3):343–56.
6. Jang YJ, Moon H. Special Consideration in the Management of Hump Noses in Asians. Facial Plast Surg 2020;36(5):554–62.
7. Bracaglia R, Tambasco D, D'Ettorre M, et al. Nougat graft": diced cartilage graft plus human fibrin glue for contouring and shaping of the nasal dorsum. Plast Reconstr Surg 2012;130(5):741e–3e.
8. Daniel RK. Diced cartilage grafts in rhinoplasty surgery: current techniques and applications. Plast Reconstr Surg 2008;122(6):1883–91.
9. Daniel RK, Calvert JW. Diced cartilage grafts in rhinoplasty surgery. Plast Reconstr Surg 2004;113(7): 2156–71.
10. Gordon CR, Alghoul M, Goldberg JS, et al. Diced cartilage grafts wrapped in AlloDerm for dorsal nasal augmentation. J Craniofac Surg 2011;22(4): 1196–9.
11. Tasman AJ. Replacement of the Nasal Dorsum with a Diced Cartilage Glue Graft. Facial Plast Surg 2019;35(1):53–7.
12. Jang YJ, Moon H. Special Consideration in Rhinoplasty for Deformed Nose of East Asians. Facial Plast Surg Clin North Am 2021;29(4):611–24.
13. Sykes JM, Kim JE, Shaye D, et al. The importance of the nasal septum in the deviated nose. Facial Plast Surg 2011;27(5):413–21.
14. Kim DY, Nam SH, Alharethy SE, et al. Surgical Outcomes of Bony Batten Grafting to Correct Caudal Septal Deviation in Septoplasty. JAMA Facial Plast Surg 2017;19(6):470–5.
15. Chen YY, Kim SA, Jang YJ. Centering a Deviated Nose by Caudal Septal Extension Graft and Unilaterally Extended Spreader Grafts. Ann otology, rhinology, Laryngol 2020;129(5):448–55.
16. Jang YJ, Sinha V. Spreader graft in septo-rhinoplasty. Indian J Otolaryngol head neck Surg 2007; 59(2):100–2.
17. Park JH, Jin HR. Use of autologous costal cartilage in Asian rhinoplasty. Plast Reconstr Surg 2012; 130(6):1338–48.
18. Won TB. Hump Nose Correction in Asians. Facial Plast Surg Clin North Am 2018;26(3):357–66.
19. Jang YJ, Yeo NK, Wang JH. Cutting and suture technique of the caudal septal cartilage for the management of caudal septal deviation. Arch Otolaryngology–Head Neck Surg 2009;135(12):1256–60.
20. Jang YJ, Kim SA, Alharethy S. Failure of Synthetic Implants: Strategies and Management. Facial Plast Surg 2018;34(3):245–54.
21. Kim SH, Kim JW, Jang YJ. Radiologic Findings of Complicated Alloplastic Implants in the Nasal Dorsum. Clin Exp Otorhinolaryngol 2021;14(3): 321–7.
22. Yu MS, Jang YJ. Preoperative computer simulation for Asian rhinoplasty patients: analysis of accuracy and patient preference. Aesthet Surg J 2014;34(8): 1162–71.
23. Jang YJ, Moon BJ. State of the art in augmentation rhinoplasty: implant or graft? Curr Opin Otolaryngol Head Neck Surg 2012;20(4):280–6.
24. Swanepoel PF, Fysh R. Laminated dorsal beam graft to eliminate postoperative twisting complications. Arch Facial Plast Surg 2007;9(4):285–9.
25. Choi WR, Jang YJ. Reconstruction of a Severely Damaged Cartilaginous Septum with a Bypass L-Strut Graft using Costal Cartilage. Facial Plast Surg : FPS 2021;37(1):92–7.

1. Publication Title	2. Publication Number	3. Filing Date
FACIAL PLASTIC SUREGERY CLINICS OF NORTH AMERICA	013 – 122	9/18/2022

4. Issue Frequency	5. Number of Issues Published Annually	6. Annual Subscription Price
FEB, MAY, AUG, NOV	4	$420.00

7. Complete Mailing Address of Known Office of Publication (Not printer) (Street, city, county, state, and ZIP+4®)

ELSEVIER INC.
230 Park Avenue, Suite 800
New York, NY 10169

Contact Person: Malathi Samayan
Telephone (Include area code): 91-44-4299-4507

8. Complete Mailing Address of Headquarters or General Business Office of Publisher (Not printer)

ELSEVIER INC.
230 Park Avenue, Suite 800
New York, NY 10169

9. Full Names and Complete Mailing Addresses of Publisher, Editor, and Managing Editor (Do not leave blank)

Publisher (Name and complete mailing address)

Stacy Eastman, ELSEVIER INC.
1600 JOHN F KENNEDY BLVD. SUITE 1800
PHILADELPHIA, PA 19103-2899

Editor (Name and complete mailing address)

Stacy Eastman ELSEVIER INC.
1600 JOHN F KENNEDY BLVD. SUITE 1800
PHILADELPHIA, PA 19103-2899

Managing Editor (Name and complete mailing address)

PATRICK MANLEY, ELSEVIER INC.
1600 JOHN F KENNEDY BLVD. SUITE 1800
PHILADELPHIA, PA 19103-2899

10. Owner (Do not leave blank. If the publication is owned by a corporation, give the name and address of the corporation immediately followed by the names and addresses of all stockholders owning or holding 1 percent or more of the total amount of stock. If not owned by a corporation, give the names and addresses of the individual owners. If owned by a partnership or other unincorporated firm, give its name and address as well as those of each individual owner. If the publication is published by a nonprofit organization, give its name and address.)

Full Name	Complete Mailing Address
WHOLLY OWNED SUBSIDIARY OF REED/ELSEVIER, US HOLDINGS	1600 JOHN F KENNEDY BLVD. SUITE 1800 PHILADELPHIA, PA 19103-2899

11. Known Bondholders, Mortgagees, and Other Security Holders Owning or Holding 1 Percent or More of Total Amount of Bonds, Mortgages, or Other Securities. If none, check box. ☑ None

Full Name	Complete Mailing Address
N/A	

12. Tax Status (For completion by nonprofit organizations authorized to mail at nonprofit rates) (Check one)
The purpose, function, and nonprofit status of this organization and the exempt status for federal income tax purposes:
☑ Has Not Changed During Preceding 12 Months
☐ Has Changed During Preceding 12 Months (Publisher must submit explanation of change with this statement)

PS Form **3526**, July 2014 [Page 1 of 4 (see instructions page 4)] PSN: 7530-01-000-9931 PRIVACY NOTICE: See our privacy policy on www.usps.com.

13. Publication Title	14. Issue Date for Circulation Data Below
FACIAL PLASTIC SUREGERY CLINICS OF NORTH AMERICA	AUGUST 2022

15. Extent and Nature of Circulation			Average No. Copies Each Issue During Preceding 12 Months	No. Copies of Single Issue Published Nearest to Filing Date
a. Total Number of Copies (Net press run)			195	180
b. Paid Circulation (By Mail and Outside the Mail)	(1)	Mailed Outside-County Paid Subscriptions Stated on PS Form 3541 (Include paid distribution above nominal rate, advertiser's proof copies, and exchange copies)	126	116
	(2)	Mailed In-County Paid Subscriptions Stated on PS Form 3541 (Include paid distribution above nominal rate, advertiser's proof copies, and exchange copies)	0	0
	(3)	Paid Distribution Outside the Mails Including Sales Through Dealers and Carriers, Street Vendors, Counter Sales, and Other Paid Distribution Outside USPS®	20	16
	(4)	Paid Distribution by Other Classes of Mail Through the USPS (e.g., First-Class Mail®)	0	0
c. Total Paid Distribution [Sum of 15b (1), (2), (3), and (4)]			146	132
d. Free or Nominal Rate Distribution (By Mail and Outside the Mail)	(1)	Free or Nominal Rate Outside-County Copies included on PS Form 3541	33	31
	(2)	Free or Nominal Rate In-County Copies Included on PS Form 3541	0	0
	(3)	Free or Nominal Rate Copies Mailed at Other Classes Through the USPS (e.g., First-Class Mail)	0	0
	(4)	Free or Nominal Rate Distribution Outside the Mail (Carriers or other means)	0	0
e. Total Free or Nominal Rate Distribution (Sum of 15d (1), (2), (3) and (4))			33	31
f. Total Distribution (Sum of 15c and 15e)			179	163
g. Copies not Distributed (See Instructions to Publishers #4 (page #3))			16	17
h. Total (Sum of 15f and g)			195	180
i. Percent Paid (15c divided by 15f times 100)			81.56%	80.98%

* If you are claiming electronic copies, go to line 16 on page 3. If you are not claiming electronic copies, skip to line 17 on page 3.

PS Form **3526**, July 2014 (Page 2 of 4)

16. Electronic Copy Circulation	Average No. Copies Each Issue During Preceding 12 Months	No. Copies of Single Issue Published Nearest to Filing Date
a. Paid Electronic Copies ▶		
b. Total Paid Print Copies (Line 15c) + Paid Electronic Copies (Line 16a) ▶		
c. Total Print Distribution (Line 15f) + Paid Electronic Copies (Line 16a) ▶		
d. Percent Paid (Both Print & Electronic Copies) (16b divided by 16c × 100) ▶		

☑ I certify that 50% of all my distributed copies (electronic and print) are paid above a nominal price.

17. Publication of Statement of Ownership

☑ If the publication is a general publication, publication of this statement is required. Will be printed in the NOVEMBER 2022 issue of this publication.

☐ Publication not required.

18. Signature and Title of Editor, Publisher, Business Manager, or Owner

Malathi Samayan

Malathi Samayan - Distribution Controller

Date: 9/18/2022

I certify that all information furnished on this form is true and complete. I understand that anyone who furnishes false or misleading information on this form or who omits material or information requested on the form may be subject to criminal sanctions (including fines and imprisonment) and/or civil sanctions (including civil penalties).

PS Form **3526**, July 2014 (Page 3 of 4) PRIVACY NOTICE: See our privacy policy on www.usps.com.

Moving?

Make sure your subscription moves with you!

To notify us of your new address, find your **Clinics Account Number** (located on your mailing label above your name), and contact customer service at:

Email: journalscustomerservice-usa@elsevier.com

800-654-2452 (subscribers in the U.S. & Canada)
314-447-8871 (subscribers outside of the U.S. & Canada)

Fax number: 314-447-8029

Elsevier Health Sciences Division
Subscription Customer Service
3251 Riverport Lane
Maryland Heights, MO 63043

*To ensure uninterrupted delivery of your subscription, please notify us at least 4 weeks in advance of move.

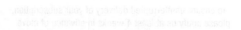

Printed and bound by CPI Group (UK) Ltd, Croydon, CR0 4YY

08/05/2025

01864723-0014